Praise for SE)

"Finally, here's a book that recognizes that most sex issues are a result of a lack of communication. Based on the latest research, *Sex Talks* helps us overcome the myths that drag us down. Buy this book! Have these essential conversations!"

—John Gottman,
New York Times bestselling author of
The Seven Principles for Making Marriage Work

"This book redefines what it means to have great sex. With her signature frankness and relatability, Vanessa Marin reveals the secrets to a fulfilling love life. You'll never think about intimacy and desire the same way again."

—Logan Ury,
author of *How to Not Die Alone:*
The Surprising Science That Will Help You Find Love

"If there's one thing I know from my years as a sex therapist, it's that talking about sex may be one of the most difficult hurdles couples face when they want to improve their sex lives. *Sex Talks* shows you how to make those conversations easier, and perhaps even fun."

—Dr. Bat Sheva Marcus,
author of *Satisfaction Guaranteed:*
How to Have the Sex You've Always Wanted

"Compassionate and witty, Marin makes what many find a challenging discussion manageable, even for readers with little idea of where to start. Anyone looking to improve their communication with a partner will find valuable takeaways."

—*Publishers Weekly*

SEX
TALKS

The Five Conversations
That Will Transform Your Love Life

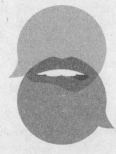

VANESSA MARIN, LMFT
with XANDER MARIN

SIMON
ELEMENT

New York   London   Toronto   Sydney   New Delhi

SIMON
ELEMENT

An Imprint of Simon & Schuster, Inc.
1230 Avenue of the Americas
New York, NY 10020

First Simon Element trade paperback edition January 2024

SIMON ELEMENT is a trademark of Simon & Schuster, Inc.

Simon & Schuster: Celebrating 100 Years of Publishing in 2024

For information about special discounts for bulk purchases, please contact Simon &
Schuster Special Sales at 1-866-506-1949 or business@simonandschuster.com.

The Simon & Schuster Speakers Bureau can bring authors to your live event. For
more information or to book an event, contact the Simon & Schuster Speakers
Bureau at 1-866-248-3049 or visit our website at www.simonspeakers.com.

Manufactured in the United States of America

1 3 5 7 9 10 8 6 4 2

Library of Congress Cataloging-in-Publication Data has been applied for.

ISBN 978-1-6680-0001-4
ISBN 978-1-6680-0931-4 (pbk)
ISBN 978-1-6680-0002-1 (ebook)

Names and identifying characteristics of some individuals
have been changed. Some dialogue has been re-created.

This book is dedicated to you, for having the courage to pick it up in the first place.

CONTENTS

INTRODUCTION

"I DON'T EVEN know what to say."

My first couples therapy session was not off to a great start. It had taken a Herculean effort to get my boyfriend, Xander, to agree to come, and to be honest, I wasn't exactly excited to be there, either. Neither one of us wanted to acknowledge the problems we were having in our relationship, and the $200 price tag didn't help. I quickly calculated that every minute I spent stumbling over my words in front of a stranger in her cramped San Francisco office cost four dollars, and I mentally lambasted myself for not figuring out what I wanted to say *before* the session had started.

I wanted to talk about our sex life. But I couldn't articulate the details of *what* was happening in our bedroom yet, because I was fixated on *how* Xander and I had gotten ourselves into such a bad place.

It had all felt so easy in the beginning. The night we met, we spent six entire hours making out, and I could have spent six more. Once we started having sex, it was a daily event (sometimes multiple times a day). Xander would get turned on by watching me stretch my arms over my head. I would get full-body shivers if he wiggled a single eyebrow at me. The chemistry between the two of us had been so undeniable I took it as a crystal-clear sign from the universe that this was my person.

But just a few short years later, everything was different. I couldn't tell you the last time we'd made out with even one-tenth the passion of our first night. We weren't having much sex, and when we did, it felt . . . vaguely disappointing? I wanted *more* from Xander, but I couldn't tell you what, exactly, that meant. I found myself feeling increasingly shy around him, like our physical intimacy had morphed from a sexy secret to a shameful one. I turned everything into a clandestine test. Would he notice me if I stepped out of the shower naked and dripping wet? How long would he go without initiating sex if I didn't ask for it first? I used to feel like I had won the soulmate lottery, but in especially lonely, quiet moments, I caught myself wondering if there was someone else out there who might be a better fit.

Although it was a deeply painful experience at the time, there's nothing extraordinary about our story. It's actually a frighteningly common one. Most couples in long-term relationships will tell you that the spark died a long time ago. We almost *expect* it to happen. Yet we still feel profoundly confused when it does.

How—and why!—does sex get so damned complicated? Why is sex so difficult to talk about, even with the person you love? Why was it even necessary for you to pick up this book in the first place?

Why People Say Talking About Sex Is Hard

We asked our Instagram community, "What holds you back from talking about sex in your relationship?" These are just a handful of the thousands of responses we received:

"I don't want to hurt her feelings."

"I don't want to make it weird."

"I feel stupid, shy, timid, awkward, and clueless. The whole thing feels taboo."

"Being truly seen."

"Not knowing what I want. I only know that I *don't* want what my partner currently does."

"Having to admit that I've been faking."

"The fear of rejection."

"My partner says we shouldn't have to talk about it; it should just happen."

"I don't want to seem needy or selfish."

"I worry I'll be misunderstood."

"I feel embarrassed, even though my partner is begging me to open up."

"I don't want her to feel pressure."

"The fear I make up in my head about his possible responses."

"I hate being vulnerable."

"Shame."

"I feel the need to protect his ego. I don't want to make him feel inadequate."

"The time never feels right."

"The fear of being judged."

"I worry that I'm letting her down."

"We just don't."

Perhaps the better question to start with is, "Why would we ever think talking about sex would be *easy?*"

Whether from your family, religion, peers, culture, or a delightful combination of the above, you were taught that sex is something to be ashamed about. That there is a specific set of rules you must abide by—with damning consequences if you don't. That sex is something that happens behind closed bedroom doors and is not to be talked about openly.

If you were lucky, the "sex education" you got took place in a sweaty eighth-grade gymnasium and involved having the bejesus scared out of you about genital warts and teenage pregnancy. No one ever taught you how to politely ask your partner to spank your ass or gently request that they stop rubbing your clitoris like they're trying to scrub a stain out of their favorite T-shirt. Or what a clitoris even is in the first place.

You almost certainly don't have any positive role models, or even examples. Despite seeing thousands of sex scenes on TV and in the movies (and probably in porn), I bet you can't pinpoint a single instance when the characters actually *talked* about what they were doing in a meaningful way. (No, J.Lo's instructing Ben Affleck to "gobble gobble" in *Gigli* doesn't count.) Instead, sex always seems like something that "just happens."

It's not like the things you need to communicate about are easy or straightforward, either. How do you tell your partner that the way they give oral sex makes your stomach turn—in a bad way—but you don't know what technique you want them to use instead? How are you supposed to know how to tell the person you love the most in this world that you're so touched out by the pressures of motherhood that you'll scream if they lay a single fingertip on you?

When I trace back through my own history with sex and communication, it makes perfect sense that I landed in that therapist's office. My version of "the talk" took place in my family's forest-green minivan after dinner at Grandma's. I saw my mom glance over at my dad, then peer at me in the rearview mirror. She practically whispered, "If you have any questions about . . . you know . . . *sex* . . . you can ask us."

I had a lot of questions. I had just made a bet at the playground with my friend Nick about the number of holes that ladies had "down there." (I confidently bet two, and lost a dollar to Nick the next day.) I wanted to know if a man had to use his hand to put his penis into a woman, or if it got sucked in there like a strong magnet. I was still picturing sex as a woman lying down on top of a man and taking a nap, and I couldn't quite understand the appeal.

But even as an awkward twelve-year-old, I knew what my parents were actually saying in that moment was, "Please, for the love of God, do not ask us *anything* about sex!" I could feel their shame and embarrassment, and I absorbed it into my own body.

Instead, I found something else to give me my sex education: women's magazines. Poring over the glossy pages, I learned that physical intimacy is what keeps men happy, so I should make sure to seem ready and willing at all times. But not *too* eager, because that would make me seem like a "slut." I read that there were certain sexual positions I needed to avoid in order to protect my partner from seeing my dreaded "belly bulge." I discovered that sneezes are like mini orgasms, so I should sneak a dash of pepper underneath a guy's nose to intensify his climax. (Side note: this is the *worst* sex advice I have ever seen. Please do not pepper your partner's nose during sex—or ever.) I had questions about the tip to put a donut over a man's penis and sexily nibble it off, but who was I to doubt the wisdom of these magazines? Most important, I learned that sex was not something you ever talked about with your partner. I was just supposed to surprise him with all these creative tricks and techniques.

Needless to say, I suffered my fair share of challenges once I became sexually active. I faked orgasms for ten years because I couldn't bring myself to talk to a partner about what I liked. I had sex I didn't really want to have because I felt too awkward to say, "No thanks, Buckaroo." I found myself on that therapist's couch, dangerously close to losing the love of my life because I couldn't tell him what I needed.

Throughout all of it, I felt deeply alone, as if I were the only person struggling to have a great sex life—much less talk about it. That's what shame does: it isolates us.

Years later, after becoming a psychotherapist myself and working with thousands of people, I finally discovered the real culprit behind the demise of Xander's and my sex life—and of yours. The loss of the spark isn't actually about the loss of the spark. It's about the lack of *communication*. Decades of work in the sex therapy field taught me that there are plenty of perfectly understandable—and more important, fixable—reasons why sex starts to feel so tricky in a relationship. But we're all struggling to talk about sex, and this lack of conversation, of even basic acknowledgment, is slowly poisoning our intimacy.

Xander and I have come a long way since our rough start, and we'll share our story with you throughout the pages of this book. But I'll give you a preview of what's to come: I've never had a relationship in which I talked about sex as openly, honestly, or frequently as I now do with Xander. I've also never had a relationship in which the sex was as deeply intimate and wildly satisfying as it is now. I don't think those two things are coincidences.

So, that's what *Sex Talks* is about: bringing sex out of the shadows, providing you with the step-by-step framework for the most crucial conversations that every couple needs to have, and giving you the courage and inspiration to open your mouth. (For *talking*!)

In the first section, you'll get to know *yourself* better, and we'll create a User Manual that you'll eventually share with your partner. In the next section, we'll cover the five elements of a truly extraordinary sex life: Acknowledgment, Connection, Desire, Pleasure, and Exploration. After testing and refining my communication techniques with thousands of people, I've learned that these are the five areas that couples struggle with the most. Then we'll wrap up with surprising techniques for keeping the spark alive for a lifetime.

You're going to learn how to politely ask for the ass spanking you've always wanted. But you're also going to discover how to create a kind of intimacy you never even dreamed possible. This book isn't a bunch of the same old recycled sex tips. No penis donuts here! Instead, *Sex Talks* is a complete paradigm shift. It gives you the crucial information you were never taught about sex, and it dives deep into some of the most complex and harmful dynamics that plague modern-day couples. You'll learn how to share your findings with your partner in a gentle yet effective way that increases intimacy and brings the two of you back home to each other. And you'll discover that the best thing you can do for your sex life doesn't even involve taking off your clothes.

The Other Half with Xander: Hi!

Throughout *Sex Talks*, I'll be jumping in to provide my perspective and share some of my experiences, because I've been on a journey of my own when it comes to communication and sex.

When Vanessa and I first met in 2007, I thought her career aspirations were pretty cool (who wouldn't want to tell their guy friends that the girl they're dating is going to be a sex therapist?). It was fun to engage with Vanessa intellectually about sex therapy as a career path, but the idea of turning the focus inward—looking at my relationship with Vanessa and my own sexuality—felt scary and way too vulnerable for a guy who "had his shit together" and "knew what he was doing in the bedroom" (i.e., the way I wanted to see myself). After all, sex therapy seemed like something only people with "real issues" needed.

And then, a few years later, Vanessa and I were having those very real problems ourselves. I was putting in sixty-plus hours a week at my job. I desperately wanted to be working less, but it felt like the only way to repay the company for the two rapid promotions I had just received was to keep saying yes to more projects. In the meantime, a combination of stress eating and complete lack of physical activity had started to reveal a figure in the mirror I didn't even recognize. In the little free time I did have, all I wanted to do was sit on the couch and watch TV. To be honest, I didn't even notice that my sex drive had disappeared until Vanessa started dropping hints that we weren't having much sex. It felt like a dagger to my heart. Like I was failing "as a man"—a man who was supposed to simultaneously have everything together and not ask for help if he didn't.

After months and months of burying my head in the sand and trying to convince myself (and Vanessa) that things would somehow improve without actually making any real change in my life, it began to dawn on me that I had a choice to make. I could continue down the path I was on and likely lose the love of my life, or I could admit I didn't have the answers and ask for some help.

So, I swallowed my pride and started therapy. Slowly but surely, I learned to get more in touch with my body, my needs, and my emotions. To allow myself to sit in the discomfort of my feelings instead of pushing them down. To set and enforce boundaries at work and in my personal life that would decrease stress. Eventually, I walked away from a career in tech that looked perfect on paper but made me feel miserable inside. And ultimately, I joined Vanessa to become the COO of the online sex therapy business she was building.

For the next few years, Vanessa begged me to get more involved with her on social media and in the courses we sold. But I was convinced I had nothing of value to share. That no one would want to hear my untrained opinions on sex and communication. Fortunately, she kept at me and encouraged me to start sharing short anecdotes and experiences from our relationship. And what I slowly came to realize is that I'm actually uniquely qualified to offer a different perspective—that of a regular dude with no psychotherapy training. A guy who has worked through his own issues with gender stereotypes and insecurities, and who has developed emotional, relational, and communication skills that have resulted in a relationship and sex life beyond my wildest dreams. I'm here to show you that you don't need a graduate degree or a clinical license to have extraordinary communication skills; you just need to have an open mind and a willingness!

What's in Store for You

Here's what I want for you during this journey:

- To feel fully seen and understood. Like, "Holy crap, Vanessa, have you been bugging my bedroom? That's *exactly* what I've been thinking/feeling/experiencing."
- To let go of any shame you may have felt about your struggles in the bedroom. I want you to know that every person and every couple struggles with sex in one way or another—Xander and myself included!
- To understand your blockages and approach them with more sensitivity and compassion.
- To level up your confidence in an authentic way.
- To laugh. Sex doesn't need to be so serious all the time! A little laughter goes a long way toward helping us all get more comfortable with our clothes off. (Plus, we're going to be sharing some ridiculous stories with you!)
- To feel hopeful that you can create an incredible sex life, and excited to get started.

By the end of *Sex Talks*, you'll be able to calmly and confidently talk about subjects that previously would have made your cheeks burn with embarrassment. But—spoiler alert!—the benefits go far beyond that. Learning how to talk about sex doesn't just impact your sex life; it also extends to all your other relationships—romantic, familial, and platonic! You'll know yourself so much better that you'll be able to connect with others on a more profound level. You'll find yourself confidently expressing your needs and making requests, navigating differences and boundaries as if you'd been in therapy for decades. And you'll believe at your very core that you deserve love, respect, connection, and intimacy.

Xander and I will be there with you every step of the way, cheering you on and helping you realize that you're much braver and more capable than you even realized! Together as a couple, we're so enthusiastic about these five Sex Talks because we've lived through both the pains of no communication and the pleasures of great communication. We're immensely proud of you for taking this courageous step of picking up this book in the first place. We know you're capable of a truly extraordinary sex life, and we're honored and excited to show you *exactly* how to get there.

A Note About Inclusivity

In writing *Sex Talks*, we both had the intention to be as inclusive as possible. This book is meant for individuals and couples of all orientations, identities, and relationship structures, not to mention skin colors, body shapes and sizes, ability levels, socioeconomic statuses, and more. We've included stories from a diverse array of people, and we have tried to avoid gendered pronouns as much as possible. We sometimes speak to specific dynamics that can occur in relationships between cisgender (or cis) men and women, and we've called out those moments.

When we say "sex" we mean it in the broadest sense of the word: anything that you do with your bodies that brings you pleasure. "Sex" is whatever it means and looks like in your life. Too often, "sex" and "intercourse" are used interchangeably, which is heteronormative and unhelpful even for male-female pairings. (We'll get into that in Conversation 4.)

Inclusivity is one of our core values—both as individuals and as a business. We firmly believe that everyone is deserving of hot sex and deep love. We know that our attempts at inclusivity will never, ever be perfect, so we are always striving to learn more and do better.

We also want to acknowledge the immense number of privileges we experience, and the filter they create in the way we see the world. We're both cis, able, financially secure, multiethnic people who are often mistaken for white. Xander is hetero and Vanessa is hetero-ish. There are so many aspects of the human experience that we will never be able to understand, despite our best intentions and efforts.

While our goal is to create and share tools that will work for as many people as possible, we know that a lot of our tips won't work for everyone. Some ideas may be downright impossible for a fair number of people. Our wish is that you find at least one nugget of wisdom in this book that helps you have the sex life you deserve!

SEX TALKS

Part One

ALL
ABOUT
YOU

CHAPTER 1

DESTROYING THE FUCKING FAIRY TALE

"DO YOU THINK there's any hope for us?" Francesca's voice breaks as she struggles to get the words out. "I love him so much. I can't imagine life without him. But I also can't continue like this."

Francesca is one of my oldest and best friends, and her husband, Jake, is a real gem of a human being, too. They're both warm, generous, intelligent, and regularly bring me to the brink of peeing in my pants from laughing so hard. Their love story is classic. They were set up by a mutual friend ("in a land before dating apps," Francesca likes to say), and their marathon blind date at a tiny Italian trattoria only came to an end when the staff politely kicked them out. Francesca and Jake gracefully slid past every milestone: becoming exclusive, getting engaged and then married, and having two beautiful and mischievous children.

Things seemed perfect from the outside, but if you looked closely, you could see signs of cracking in the façade. Francesca had a certain way she liked to do things around the house and would get over-the-top irritated at Jake for messing up the pantry organization or folding the towels "like a heathen." Jake tended to withdraw, retreating to the basement to watch his beloved Packers and losing himself in long hours at his law firm. The raucous date nights they had once cherished became increasingly infrequent, especially once they became parents.

Francesca and Jake's sex life had grown more complicated, too. At the beginning of their relationship, Francesca and I would spend entire brunches dissecting every last detail of their wildly passionate bedroom escapades. But over time, Francesca's bragging turned into venting. She disclosed that she rarely initiated sex; even though she considered herself a feminist, she still had the nagging feeling that it should be up to the guy to make it happen. Unbeknownst to Jake, Francesca had been faking orgasms with increasing frequency over the years. Her performance had become half-hearted, and she was growing resentful of him for rolling off her right after having his own climax. ("Sometimes I don't even bother to fake an orgasm," she tells me, "but he still seems to think that once *he's* done, *we're* done.")

Separately, Jake confided in me that Francesca sometimes seemed disinterested and distant during sex, and he would lose his erection in those moments. He'd catch himself feeling anxious the next time they started taking their clothes off, wondering if he was going to be able to stay hard.

Their frequency had dropped to maybe a fourth of what it was at the beginning of their relationship, and their satisfaction was at an all-time low.

A Category 5 stress hurricane pushed everything to the surface. In a single week, their daughter broke her leg during gymnastics practice, their roof sprung a massive leak, and Jake got passed over for a promotion he'd been gunning for. The tension was palpable for days, and by Friday night, Francesca and Jake were looking forward to the moment they could finally relax. After the kids were asleep, they poured glasses of wine, crawled into bed, and turned on a movie. Francesca was just starting to drift off to sleep when Jake started rubbing her back. She tensed up immediately; she knew what his "massage" meant—but couldn't Jake see that his timing was ridiculously bad? Francesca whined, "J, I'm *exhausted.*" Jake rolled over onto his side of the bed, letting out a dramatic sigh. His obvious disappointment set Francesca off in a way she had never before experienced.

"How could you be thinking of sex at a time like this?" Francesca snarled at him.

"Because I can't even remember the last time we had sex!" Jake huffed back.

The fight still had Francesca rattled on our walk the next morning. "I don't really know what to do," Francesca says. "I mean, he's right. I can't remember the last time we had sex, either." She takes a deep breath, and her voice goes soft and quiet. "It shouldn't be this hard, should it?"

"Should we really get into it?" I ask. "Or did you just want to vent?"

"I need you in full-blown sex therapist mode," she responds, rubbing at the bags under her eyes. "Help me fix this, please."

Understanding Why Sex Gets So Complicated

What's the first step for Francesca, for me, and for you? Understanding that the fairy-tale version of sex (and relationships) we all have in our heads is just that—a fairy tale. I like to call it the *Fucking* Fairy Tale. Just like TV and the movies lead us to believe that we'll have a meet-cute with our one true love, overcome some mild adversity, then live happily ever after, we're also fed an overly simplified version of what our sex life with said true love will be like. Hollywood sex always unfolds spontaneously and effortlessly, zero communication required. The chemistry is so intense you can practically feel it through the screen. Couples always orgasm in the same instant, from three pumps of Missionary-position intercourse, and everyone seems wildly satisfied. When I ask people to describe their ideal sex life, the most common word I hear is "natural." We *crave* that feeling of effortlessness we've witnessed on the screen countless times.

Except that's not how it unfolds in our own relationships. And that leaves us feeling confused, scared, and even angry. Francesca tells me, "I guess I'm naïve, but I didn't realize how much work relationships and sex take. Our connection was so strong at first that I assumed it would always be solid. When the spark fades, you almost resent the fact that you have to work at it, because in the movies it all looks so easy."

I know from personal experience that this transition from fairy tale to train wreck can be incredibly scary, so I run Francesca through the specific reasons we find ourselves here in the first place. Because it happens to the best of us, and it's not entirely your fault.

Blame Your Brain

Let's start with one of the most straightforward reasons chemistry with your partner feels so much stronger at the beginning of a relationship: literal chemistry. In your early months together, the neurotransmitters in your brain go buck wild. The serotonin levels there are similar to those in someone who has obsessive-compulsive disorder, and the dopamine levels mimic being high on cocaine. It's *that* intense!

But this stage can last for only one to three years, max. At that point, your previously surging high-octane transmitters—serotonin, dopamine, and norepinephrine—get replaced with oxytocin and vasopressin, which are designed to help us relax and bond. We shift into creating deeper attachment to our partner and forging a strong, secure, lasting foundation.

Brain chemistry isn't the entire picture, but it's useful to know that your brain is *physically incapable* of maintaining that same level of lust over the long term. If, like Francesca, you find yourself feeling sad and scared that it seems so much harder to be attracted to and turned on by your partner, stop judging yourself. Losing desire is actually more "natural" than feeling it constantly.

The Stress Shutdown

As soon as I mention the word "stress," Francesca rolls her eyes. "I know, I'm too stressed. But that's just life." Like most of us, Francesca has gotten used to juggling never-ending responsibilities and ever-increasing pressure. It has become her default mode of functioning—so much so that in the rare moments when she's not busy, she finds herself feeling anxious.

Most people don't realize that stress is the number one sex drive killer. When you're stressed, your body thinks that it's under attack. It goes into fight-or-flight mode, deciding whether to stay and duke it out or get the hell out of there. During those moments, your system releases a hormone called cortisol, which shuts down unnecessary functions so you can focus all your energy on protecting yourself. Libido is one of the first things to go.

Think about our ancestors—if a caveman was being chased by a woolly mammoth, why would he also need to have an erection at the same time? If anything, a raging boner flapping around between his thighs is just going to slow him down! Cortisol is helpful if you *are* in danger in the moment, but when your body is *constantly* in that state of high tension, it basically ensures that your sex drive never kicks back into gear.

When Two Become Three, or Four, or Five

When you have children, your focus changes. Francesca and Jake used to live in their own little world together, and while their children have been a happy addition, they've also dramatically changed the balance of things. Francesca and Jake aren't each other's primary focus anymore, and their list of responsibilities has exploded. As Francesca puts it, "Jake started to feel like yet another item on the long list of people or things that need 'doing.'" Francesca also lovingly calls her kids "the greatest cockblocks of all time." The kids are always around, they manage to sneak into Francesca and Jake's bed most nights, and Francesca is usually nervous about them overhearing sex or barging in at the worst possible moment. Even when Francesca and Jake are alone, Francesca finds herself struggling to relax. She tells me, "It's like when you start working from home, sometimes it's hard to separate your work time and your leisure time . . . except with being a parent you never get to log off. There really is no place in my home that I don't feel like a parent. At least with work, your boss doesn't wake you up in the middle of the night because they had another nightmare about monsters!"

Relationship researcher John Gottman found that 67 percent of couples report that their marital satisfaction plummeted after having kids.[1] But, like most parents, Francesca and Jake are also exhausted, too busy and overwhelmed to even put much thought into repairing their relationship. Francesca tells me, "It's easier to let things slide than to address them. I'm just so tired that a difficult conversation is the last thing I want to do . . . until I realize I'm in survival mode and unsure how to move forward with someone who's a roommate with whom I'm raising kids."

The Pain of Rejection

At the beginning of a relationship, it feels easy to say yes to everything. You agree to all date-night ideas, even the ones that feel a little out of your comfort zone. You take your partner up on most of their invitations to have sex. It feels like you have all this good energy and momentum propelling you forward.

That all comes to a screeching halt when the word "no" enters your relationship vocabulary. I want to be perfectly clear in saying that you are always allowed to say no—to anything, for whatever reason.

Rejection is a normal and healthy part of every relationship, but the problem is that none of us are prepared for it. Hearing the word "no" from our partner, especially when it comes to sex, typically brings up enormous amounts of shame. I have memories seared into my brain of Xander turning me down for sex, and the feelings of embarrassment and even humiliation that overcame me in those moments. Rejection feels so terrible that most of us will go to great lengths to avoid it. If your partner turns you down, your instinct is likely to stop initiating. But if no one is initiating, what do you think is going to happen to your sex life?

Performance Issues

Our bodies aren't machines, and they don't always do what we want them to do. It's normal to experience a dry vulva, a soft penis, or an orgasm that's too fast or takes too long. (And stress can make all these issues so much worse, too.) But performance issues definitely aren't part of the Fucking

Fairy Tale, so that leaves us feeling like it's yet another thing we can't talk about openly.

Great Sexpectations: Sexual Perfectionism

The Fucking Fairy Tale expectations of sex affect us on a relationship level, but also on an individual one. In the Hollywood version of sex, everyone knows what they're doing, and they look sexy doing it. No one ever has to ask for directions on how to perform varsity-level oral sex. No one ever has a pimple on their butt cheek or bits of toilet paper stuck in their labia. No one's ever thinking about their grocery list while being ravaged by their partner. It leaves us feeling like we have to be just as polished in the bedroom—a phenomenon I call Sexual Perfectionism. It's the desire to control every aspect of an interaction so that you seem flawless to your partner and to yourself.

If you can't talk about sex in your relationship, Sexual Perfectionism takes a dangerously strong hold on you. As we walk our dogs on the beach, Xander tells me about how this happened for him early in our relationship: "I didn't feel comfortable talking about sex, so the stakes felt so much higher. I felt like I had to be perfect at sex so that there would never be anything for you to say about it. But no one ever taught me what it means to be 'good at sex,' so I turned to movies and porn."

Sexual Perfectionism leaves no room for the intricacies of being human, and it tells us that physical intimacy needs to fit an exacting set of standards. Here are some of the ways my clients have described their expectations of sex:

"I should be able to get turned on spontaneously and easily."
"I should have a hot body that looks incredible in every position."
"I should be confident, wild, and uninhibited."
"Every time I try something new, it should happen exactly as I planned."

"We need to have simultaneous orgasms every time."

"I should satisfy my partner and be the best they've ever had."

(Pro tip: Anytime you hear yourself saying the word "should," you're probably veering into perfectionism territory. I had a great professor in grad school who used to tell me, "Vanessa, stop shoulding all over yourself.")

For Francesca, perfectionism takes the form of being too afraid to initiate. She had tried to be more assertive with a previous partner, but he laughed at her and called her awkward. So, she's extremely hesitant to initiate sex with Jake. In addition to her fears of not being sexy enough with her technique, she worries about how rejected she'd feel if Jake said he wasn't in the mood. "I'm already self-conscious enough about my mom belly. If he said no to me, I would take it so personally. Like it would be confirmation that he's not attracted to me anymore, and he wishes I had my old body back."

My story is different from Francesca's, but I can relate. I spent years chasing my individual version of the Fucking Fairy Tale. I wanted to be perfectly sexy and confident, seducing my partner with every look and touch. I fixated on my partner's experience and ignored my own, trying to give them the impression that we were "clicking" during sex. I faked pleasure, faked orgasm, faked pretty much everything. All in the service of Sexual Perfectionism.

But my performance wasn't good for anyone, and I doubt yours is, either. Sexual Perfectionism leads to sex that is high on awkwardness and pressure, and low on enjoyment and intimacy. It even chips away at your sex drive: Why would you crave such an anxiety-inducing experience?

But perhaps the worst side effect of Sexual Perfectionism is that it leaves you stuck. You're unsatisfied with your non-fairy-tale sex life, bored of repeating the exact same routine, but you're also too self-conscious to suggest or start something different. We all want to see ourselves as someone who is "great at sex," so we stick with what we know out of the fear that if we try something new, it won't go perfectly. The devil you know is better than the devil you don't, right?

But in this book, I'm asking you—and your partner—to step outside your comfort zone, be vulnerable, and take some risks, so we've got to work together to overcome your Sexual Perfectionism.

The Other Half with Xander: Normalizing the Imperfections

Most people assume Vanessa and I have the perfect sex life. Like we're always horny, constantly trying new things, and having earth-shattering orgasms every time. Sometimes everything comes together and we have truly exceptional sex, but oftentimes it's far from ideal.

In fact, here's what sex looked like for Vanessa and me just last week. I initiated by casually mumbling, "Wanna do it?" (Note to self: You gotta stop saying this!) Vanessa gave me the side-eye in response, so it was pretty clear she would have appreciated a more enthusiastic invitation. Once we got started, my erection wasn't as rock hard as it can sometimes be, and I found myself worrying at times about losing it. Vanessa wasn't particularly wet when we started having intercourse, and I got distracted wondering if I should grab the lube from the nightstand. We had an awkward dirty talk situation when I didn't quite catch something Vanessa said and responded with a loud "What?!" Overall, there were moments when things felt really good, and moments when things felt a little flat or off. My orgasm was all right, but I've definitely had better. We got some bodily fluids on the sheets that had just been washed. And afterward, Vanessa wanted to get up and do something together, but I was tired and wanted to stay in bed for a few minutes to collect myself.

Despite all that, both Vanessa and I still enjoyed the experience, because our expectations of sex aren't sky high. Neither of us needs or wants unwavering perfection in each and every moment. Of course, if either one of us is having a negative or unpleasurable experience, we take action and either change things up ourselves or make a request of each other. But if we're just experiencing minor ups and downs, we let it be, and we definitely don't dwell on it afterward. Just giving ourselves that permission allows us to better enjoy the experience.

This is what sex in the real world looks like. It's not effortless. It's not spontaneous. It involves zero mind reading. It's awkward, messy, and, quite frankly, kinda bizarre. We all fart. We queef. Sometimes we even bump heads when we switch positions. And that's all okay! Seriously.

Plus, if we did have "perfect" sex every time, that would become "normal" and there wouldn't be any exceptional times to appreciate!

Releasing the Pressure

After Francesca and I talk about the Fucking Fairy Tale and Sexual Perfectionism, she asks me, "So, am I just supposed to resign myself to a lifetime of boring sex? Or no sex at all? On the one hand, I feel like I have zero energy for it right now. But I hate myself for that, and it feels awful to think of just throwing in the towel on our sex life."

"I'm telling you that it's not going to be perfect, *not* that it's going to be terrible!" I respond. "We have to tear down all the bullshit expectations you've been taught to have when it comes to sex. *Then* we build you back up again with a healthier outlook and approach. Sex can be passionate, pleasurable, and satisfying. But it's going to look different from the Fucking Fairy Tale."

Francesca nods.

"Okay, let's figure out how we're going to do this."

Sexual perfectionism is very personal, so the approach that works best for one person isn't going to work for another. See my favorite techniques below and choose the ones that pique your curiosity. Start with one tip at a time and come back when you feel ready for another. Repetition is the key to dismantling Sexual Perfectionism, so this is going to be a lifelong journey for most of us.

Feel Your Feels

Francesca caught my attention when she said "I hate myself for that," so I started there.

"I know you're feeling a whole lot of feelings about what's going on with you and Jake right now. You're confused, sad, upset, hopeless, anxious, and so much more. And I've heard you beat yourself up for having those emotions. So, not only are you dealing with the feelings themselves, which are challenging enough, but you're also heaping on your *feelings* about your feelings. That's just too much."

Francesca laughs. "Tell me about it."

"I want to help you break this cycle by giving yourself permission to feel whatever it is that you're feeling. Whenever you notice yourself having a thought or emotion about your sex life, tell yourself, 'Okay, I'm anxious, or frustrated, or sad, and that's all right. I don't need to criticize myself about it, too.' The best way to navigate your feelings is to simply notice them and leave them be. What we resist, persists! When we accept our own emotions and experiences, they actually dissipate much faster. That's the foundation of emotional intelligence. You think you can try that?"

"Sure," she says. "Sounds better than how I'm currently handling things. I'll just pretend you're there with me in the moment telling me, 'Ches, it's okay to feel your feels.'"

Play Out the Tape

Here's a sobering question to ask yourself: What will your sex life look like if you continue taking a perfectionistic approach to sex? This may sound dramatic, but how will you feel if you're on your deathbed, looking back at a lifetime of refusing to try new techniques, being lost in self-critical thoughts, and never experiencing true intimacy with your partner?

Examine Your Expectations

Make a list of exactly what you think you're supposed to do in the bedroom. Then take a good, hard look at it, and ask yourself if those expectations are reasonable. Would you tell your best friend that they needed to live up to those same guidelines? Sometimes taking an objective look at the expectations you have of yourself helps you realize how ridiculously high you've set your standards.

I did this exercise with my client Taron, a queer cis male still in the honeymoon stage with a new partner. Taron was suffering from horrible performance anxiety around his erection. He wrote on his list, "Get a boner as soon as I initiate." I asked him, "So, you think you should get hard with zero stimulation? You should just get an erection the instant you think to ask your partner, 'Hey, Babe, want to head up to the bedroom?' Neither you nor your partner should need to touch, kiss, lick, or stimulate your penis in *any* way?" His face blanched. "Damn," he said, "When you put it that way, it sounds ridiculous."

Identify the True Villain

If you're a perfectionist, your brain likely spews controlling and insulting thoughts at you all day long. These judgments can be so frequent and intense that you assume you're the one thinking them. But you're actually hearing the voice of your inner critic, which is just one very small part of you. If you name that villain, or even come up with a full character for them, you can distance yourself from those harsh thoughts. When you hear your inner critic jabbering away at you, talk back to them.

Francesca loved this particular tool and decided to name her inner critic Barb. The next time she caught Barb telling her she couldn't possibly initiate sex, she said to herself, "Okay, Barb, I know you're worried about looking like an idiot. But Jake hasn't ever laughed at me, and he's always telling me he wants to feel desired by me." When she noticed negative thoughts during sex, she thought, "Listen, Barb, I know you've got a thing against my stomach pooch hanging over when I'm on top, but I'm done letting you dictate my sex life."

Make a Plan

My client Petra wanted to try Cowgirl position, but she was too intimidated. She said she didn't know how to do it properly, and she was scared that her boyfriend Wesley would make fun of her if she didn't move her hips "in the right way."

Wesley was there in the session, so I turned to him.

"Do you want to try Cowgirl?" I asked.

"Yes, ma'am!" he responded, a big smile on his face.

"Do you solemnly swear that you will not laugh at Petra, even if she messes up Cowgirl in the worst possible way?"

"Absolutely!"

Sometimes it really can be as simple as that. Bring your fears out into the light of day and make a game plan for addressing the worst-case scenario.

Open Up to Your Partner

Even though we're not yet in the section of the book where you're having structured conversations with your partner, it's still a good time to think about how you might eventually talk to your partner about your fears. Can you tell your partner about the Fucking Fairy Tale version of sex that you're trying to dismantle? The Sexual Perfectionism you're battling? Can you open up about the specific fears or anxieties you have? And can you create a safe space for them to share their own struggles with you? Because I can practically guarantee you that you're not alone.

If you allow it to happen, this can be a major bonding experience for the two of you. This is what true intimacy is—letting our partner see our internal world, even when it's not a pretty picture. Not keeping our guard up, like we do with strangers.

JUST THE TIP(S):

- Fuck the Fucking Fairy Tale. Sex in the real world looks nothing like it does on TV, in the movies, or in porn.
- Sexual Perfectionism is destroying your sex life. It's putting unnecessary pressure on you and your partner, ruining your sex drive, and preventing you from getting unstuck.
- You're never going to feel like you know exactly what you're doing or have it all together. Awkwardness is the price of admission for a smoking-hot sex life.

CHAPTER 2

CREATING YOUR USER MANUAL

AALIYAH FLOPS ONTO my couch, sighing loudly as she sweeps her box braids behind her back.

"I've been ticking down the days until this session," she says. "I have so much to fill you in on."

"Oh yeah? What's up?" I respond.

"The headline: ENM is *intense*." Aaliyah practices ethical non-monogamy. She and her boyfriend, Sebastian, recently opened up their relationship, and they spent a few months in couples therapy ironing out their boundaries around how much intimacy they feel comfortable sharing with other people. Aaliyah met Bryce in a dating app tailored to open relationships, and they started having sex a few weeks ago. All these theoretical situations she and Sebastian discussed in therapy are suddenly feeling a whole lot more complicated now that she's being intimate with a real person who is not Sebastian.

"Everything with Bryce feels so different than it does with Sebastian," Aaliyah continues.

This is one of those moments in a session when I know that all I need to do to be a good therapist is to encourage her to keep talking. So, I go with the time-honored therapeutic "Hmm . . . ?"

Aaliyah takes the bait.

"I mean, obviously it would; Bryce is Bryce, and Sebastian is Sebastian. But it's throwing me for a loop. Like, with Bryce, oral feels amazing, even though I've never been that into it with Sebastian. I don't think Bryce is doing rocket science down there, so how can I enjoy it so much more with him? And I think Sebastian can sense that I'm not as into sex with him right now, and he keeps asking me what I want when we're doing it, which drives me nuts because I don't know what to tell him. I *don't know* why it feels so different."

I open my mouth, but Aaliyah isn't ready for me to say anything just yet.

"And also, I'm so horny for Bryce, in a way I don't think I ever was with Sebastian. I know, New Relationship Energy, but it feels like there's more to it than that. Like it's got me questioning my chemistry with Sebastian. I can't get enough of Bryce, but it's so much harder to get turned on for Sebastian, which breaks my heart because I love Sebastian."

The energy in the room shifts. Aaliyah slows down to catch her breath, and that's when the tears come.

"And that's not even the worst part. I feel like *I'm* a different person with each of them. The woman I am with Sebastian is not the woman who shows up with Bryce. It's like I don't really know who I am anymore."

She grabs a tissue. "I should have booked a double session, huh?" she says sarcastically.

———

Your unique situation may or may not involve multiple partners, but I'm willing to bet you can relate to a central thread running through Aaliyah's story: the feeling of being a stranger to yourself, sexually. You might feel confused about what you need in the bedroom, or why it seems to shift all the time. Or it may feel like you have no freaking clue what you want.

As you and your partner work your way through the five Sex Talks, you're going to learn a whole lot more about yourself. In preparation for having these conversations with your partner, I want to help you start building a foundation of sexual self-awareness. There are two particular topics from the five conversations that are especially useful to explore on your own first: what you need to get turned on, and what you need to enjoy yourself.

I want to acknowledge that if you're the one who picked up this book, and you're reading it alone, it may feel frustrating or even scary to turn the lens on yourself. Maybe you've been trying to get your partner to talk about your sex life for years, but they've managed to wriggle, Houdini-like, out of a conversation every time. This book may even be a last-ditch effort to save your relationship before you throw in the towel. It may be tempting to blame your partner and focus on all the ways they've gotten the two of you into this mess. But nothing in a relationship is ever just one person's "fault." And even if your partner was magically to blame for everything, and even if you were to wind up making the horribly painful decision to end the relationship, it's still going to be worth it for you to go on this personal exploration.

Plus, this process of self-discovery is going to be easier than you think. Here's the thing both Aaliyah and you need to hear: you already know more about your own desires and needs than you realize.

"Me" versus "We": The Secret to Understanding Your Libido

When I ask people to tell me their biggest frustration with their sex life, one of the most common answers is low libido. Most people have this idea in their heads of how often and how strongly they're supposed to desire sex, but feel like they're not living up to their own expectations. When we asked our Instagram audience if they wanted to have a higher sex drive, 77 percent of respondents said yes. (You'll see me reference our casual Instagram polls throughout the book. While they're certainly not scientific, we regularly get anywhere from twenty thousand to fifty thousand responses, providing some interesting data points.) After seeing that poll, a number of people messaged to say, "I *want* to want sex more, but I can't even get to that place."

Dealing with low sex drive can be emotionally painful. You might fear that something's wrong with you if your sex drive was never very high to begin with. If it decreased over time, you may worry that you'll never be able to get it back. Or you might externalize it, like Aaliyah, wondering if you're not in the right relationship or not with the right partner. (We'll get back to this in Part Two.) I've personally dealt with phases of low libido, and they left me feeling like a shell of myself. Like all my vitality and femininity had been drained out of me. I wanted to understand why I had so little desire for sex, but it felt like a puzzle I couldn't even begin to solve. Even thinking about it left me feeling exhausted.

Fortunately, we now have plenty of tools to help us understand how sex drive really works, and what it needs to stay humming. To begin with, I like to think about desire in terms of "Me" versus "We" dynamics. Some aspects of sex drive happen internally (the "Me"), and some can form between you and your partner (the "We"). We'll talk about the "We" bucket when we get to the five big conversations, but in this chapter we'll be talking about the "Me."

Identifying Your Sex Drive Type

Did you know there are two completely different types of sex drive? This is some of the most fascinating research that has come out of the field of sex therapy in the last few years, and I have to give credit where it's deserved—to Emily Nagoski—for breaking this down in her terrific book *Come as You Are*. If you want to have an active sex life, it's crucial that you identify your type. And hot damn, am I excited to share this with you. Any time I talk about the sex drive types on Instagram, I get flooded with tearful DMs from people saying things like, "I have to tell you that sex drive type info just blew my mind. For so long I thought I was broken, but now I realize I just didn't understand how my sex drive works."

There are two ways we get turned on and ready for sex: in our heads (mental desire) and in our bodies (physical arousal). Mental desire is when sex sounds good. For people with penises, physical arousal means getting an erection and the testicles tightening and lifting. For people with vaginas, it means getting lubricated. For everyone, it means nipples getting hard, heart rate increasing, breath deepening, and blood rushing to the genitals.

Most people think of desire and arousal as the same thing, and that both should happen at the same time. All of a sudden, out of nowhere, you should feel interested in sex, and your body should be perfectly ready to have it in that instant. But in reality, mental desire and physical arousal happen separately, and your sex drive type depends on where you initially feel interested in getting intimate—in your head or in your body.

If you're a Spontaneous type, you feel mental desire first, then physical arousal second.

If you're a Responsive type, you feel physical arousal first, then mental desire second.

Spontaneous desire occurs when you're just going about your day and you suddenly realize that you're mentally in the mood. When the characters in your favorite TV show have passionate, impromptu sex against the wall or in the restaurant bathroom because they can't wait another second, that's Spontaneous desire at play. You're probably a Spontaneous type if:

- You feel the desire for sex at seemingly random points throughout the day. (In the middle of a work meeting, while raking the lawn, or even on the toilet!)
- You sometimes feel the desire for sex before your body responds— as in, you're in the mood, but you don't have an erection, aren't wet, or haven't had any other physical response.
- You're typically the one who initiates sex in your relationship.
- You seem to want sex more frequently than your partner. (Key word there is "seem." More on this in a minute.)

- You can feel turned on in a lot of different situations. (When your in-laws just stopped over? No problem!)

Responsive desire is the exact opposite; it's when you get mentally turned on in response to some sort of physical stimulus. You might be watching a hot sex scene in a movie, or kissing your partner, and you notice that you're starting to tingle between your legs. Sometimes you don't feel mentally interested in sex until you've already had sex and it's over! You might have a Responsive sex drive if:

- You rarely think about sex.
- Sex doesn't sound tempting until you're getting started or in the middle of it.
- Sometimes at the end of sex, you think to yourself, "That was fun. Why don't I want that more often?"
- You rarely initiate sex with your partner.
- You seem to want sex less frequently than your partner.
- It feels like the situation needs to be "just right" in order for you to feel turned on. (The bedroom has to be tidied, the kids have to be asleep, and you have to be fresh out of the shower.)

Here's another way to sum up the two types:

SPONTANEOUS DESIRE: Feel turned on, then start having sex.
RESPONSIVE DESIRE: Start having sex, then feel turned on.

Every person can experience both types of desire, but most of us tend to be more in one camp than in the other. In general, men tend to experience Spontaneous desire more frequently, while women tend to experience Responsive desire more frequently.[1]

Most people tend to think that Spontaneous desire is better, because that's how we see it in Hollywood. If you don't feel that mental desire out of nowhere, you probably think that something is wrong with you. But the reality is that neither type of desire is better or worse than the other; they're just different.

The joy of having Spontaneous desire is that it can be a lot of fun to have sex randomly pop into your head. We have so much crap running through our minds on a daily basis, and it can be exciting to have a sexy thought instead! The joy of having Responsive desire is that it invites you to be much more connected to your body, since that's what you need to stimulate first.

Each of the two sex drive types also has its own challenges. In my clinical experience, Spontaneous sex drive types experience more performance issues than Responsive types. If you're a Spontaneous type, you can feel the mental interest in sex, but your body won't always respond. You're turned on, your partner is turned on, but you're as soft as a sea cucumber or as dry as a desert. For most people, that's a deeply humiliating experience. (It *shouldn't* be, but it often is.) And your partner might take it personally, worrying that it's a sign you're not attracted to them.

If you're a Responsive sex drive type, you have completely different struggles, mainly stemming from the fact that most people don't realize this type of desire exists. It probably seems to you and your partner that you rarely—or even never—want sex. But that's just not true! You're not low desire; you just need to feel physically aroused *first*, and then your mental desire will follow. Your desire is going to show itself when you give it something to respond to. So, you need to rejigger your expectations about the order of events when you're having sex with your partner. Allow yourself to start getting physical first (in a way that feels safe; we'll get to this later), then see if that leads to you wanting more.

Let's pause for a moment here.

- What sex drive type do you think you have?
- What type do you think your partner has?
- How have both of your types affected your relationship?

In a session with Aaliyah, we discovered that both she and Sebastian are primarily Responsive types, while Bryce is a tried-and-true Spontaneous. Aaliyah and Bryce did have the New Relationship Energy going for them, but Bryce's Spontaneous desire also played a role in making their sex life feel extra exciting. Bryce would take the lead in initiating intimacy, since his Spontaneous drive made him think of it more frequently. He would get Aaliyah's Responsive desire fired up by giving her massages or making out with her for long periods of time. Sebastian and Aaliyah, with their identical types, would often wait for the other to initiate. Sex could often feel like a stand-off, with both of them hoping their partner would take the lead and get the party started. Aaliyah had been afraid that her waning sex life with Sebastian was a sign that they weren't a great fit, especially in comparison to Bryce. But once she understood the role their sex drive types were playing, she had her own "hot damn" moment.

Getting to Know What Turns You . . . Off

As soon as Aaliyah understands the Responsive issue with Sebastian, she immediately asks, "So, how do I feel hornier for Sebastian?"

It's the question most people have when they're struggling with low sex drive. We all want to know that one simple trick that will magically get us fired up. Is there a magic pill? Supplements? Oysters? Chocolate? Or my favorite: "I saw some influencer on Instagram sharing about a crystal you put under your pillow at night. . . . Does that really work?" (The answer to all of the above is a resounding no.)

I'll give you practical tips for getting turned on. But there's something else we have to explore first. You see, early in my sex therapy career, I gave my clients plenty of advice for getting their sex drives revving, but they kept coming back week after week, telling me that nothing was working. "I just feel like I'm hitting a brick wall," one of my clients complained. And that's when it dawned on me: We have to get our libidos out of Reverse before we can go into Drive, just like you need to back out of your driveway before you can cruise down the street. I started testing this theory with my clients, and it proved to be far more successful.

Getting Out of Reverse

Think about a recent time that your partner initiated sex but you weren't in the mood. Try to remember as many details of that moment as you can. Then, think about these questions:

- Was there anything about that specific situation that made you disinterested in sex?
- Was there anything you did (purposely or accidentally) that turned you off?
- Was there anything your partner did (purposely or accidentally) that put you into Reverse?

Consider things that happened in the moment itself and the dynamics that came up long before sex even got initiated. In Part Two, I'm going to give you a powerful reframe for the moment that sex actually gets started. Hint: it's not when clothes come off, and it's not even when sex gets initiated. Here are some possibilities:

I was tired.

I was afraid I would be in pain during sex.

I was full.

My partner initiated sex in a way that I didn't like.

I was intoxicated.

I was worried about my appearance.

I felt stressed or pressured.

I was anxious about my performance.

I was focused on other things, like the kids or my to-do list.

I was unhappy with my partner.

I felt guilty or ashamed about sex.

I was worried about pregnancy or STIs.

I knew I wouldn't enjoy the sex that we would have.

I was sick.

I was triggered by memories of past sexual abuse I've experienced.

I didn't know how to ask my partner for what I wanted, or I didn't know what I wanted in the first place.

I was depressed or anxious.

There wasn't enough privacy.

I was dealing with an injury.

There wasn't enough time.

Repeat this exercise the next few times you're not in the mood, and see what themes start to emerge.

Finally, take a look at your answers and think about these questions:

- What are the three most frequent dynamics that typically put you in Reverse?
- What are the three most powerful things you or your partner could do to prevent you from going into Reverse?

Sexual Pain and Your Libido

According to the April 2015 issue of the *Journal of Sexual Medicine*, 30 percent of women experienced pain during their last sexual encounter.[2] Yes, you read that right: 30 percent!

Pain is not only unpleasant in the moment; it also annihilates your desire to have sex in the first place. Our bodies are hardwired to avoid pain. Do you ever wonder why you don't feel wildly turned on by the idea of putting your hand on a hot stove or throwing yourself down a flight of stairs? Of course not! So, why would you think sex would be any different? It sounds obvious when I lay it out like that, but many women don't make that connection.

If you're struggling with painful sex, here are some changes you can try:

- Use lube every single time.
- Give yourself at least fifteen minutes to warm up and get aroused before attempting any sort of penetration.
- Go slow with any in-and-out movements, especially at first.
- Experiment with different positions and angles to see what feels most comfortable for your body.
- Get regular check-ups with your OB/GYN.
- See a pelvic pain specialist or pelvic floor physical therapist if you suspect you have a bigger issue.
- *Do not* force yourself to endure painful sex! You'll create a dissociative relationship with your body and may even build up resentment toward your partner.

Aaliyah's Reverse dynamics become evident to her quickly. "It's always when it's late at night and I'm beat. It's not gonna happen after a big meal. Or when I'm wearing my raggedy nightshirt to bed, because I never feel sexy in that old thing. If Sebastian's been farting, that's an immediate no from me. So, some low-hanging fruit would be to have sex earlier in the day, buy cuter jammies, and ask Sebastian to clench them cheeks."

At the end of the session, she muses, "This *is* a whole lot more complicated than Sebastian just not being the right partner for me. It's annoying to realize that a lot of this is on me, but I guess I'm also kinda glad you're pushing me to do this exploration. I *am* getting to know myself better."

Now that you've gotten yourself out of Reverse, let's talk about getting into Drive.

Getting to Know What Turns You On

I ask Aaliyah to think about a recent time with Sebastian when she *did* feel in the mood, and to consider the situation, her own actions, and Sebastian's actions. The answers don't come as quickly for Aaliyah as they did with her Reverse dynamics, which is common. For most people it's a lot easier to think about your turn-*offs* (ugh, the farts!) than your turn-*ons*.

So, I assign her a tracking exercise and ask her to spend two weeks paying closer attention to anything that even remotely inched her toward Drive. I tell her to think about each of her five senses. What types of sights, sounds, smells, tastes, and touches turn her on?

I also tell Aaliyah to imagine that she gets offered $100,000 to write an erotic novel. She doesn't have to actually write it, but I wanted her to daydream about what her story arc would be, and what individual sex scenes would look like. (There's something about imagining getting paid money for this that makes the exercise so much more powerful for my clients!)

Finally, I warn Aaliyah that her Drive dynamics are going to be all over the place in terms of effort required. Some will seem like simple and immediate changes that she could make, like having sex before eating. (I'll share the game-changing Fuck First rule later!) And some dynamics will take more time and energy to address, such as working on improving her body image or processing religious guilt.

"Your sex drive is a lifelong project, so don't get discouraged!" I tell her. "Any effort that you put into minimizing your Reverses and maximizing your Drives will make an impact."

Getting into Drive

Think about a recent time that you *did* feel in the mood for sex. Try to remember as many details as you can. Here are some questions to consider:

- Was there anything about the situation that helped you feel interested in sex?
- Was there anything you did (purposely or accidentally) that turned you on?
- Was there anything your partner did (purposely or accidentally) that put you into Drive?
- What types of sights, sounds, smells, tastes, and touches turn you on?

Again, think about dynamics that happened in the moment and long before sex got started.

Here are some possibilities:

I had energy.

I felt confident.

My partner had done their fair share of work for our household/family.

I enjoyed the way my partner initiated, or the way I initiated.

I wanted to connect with my partner.

My partner and I felt connected
before we started getting physical.

I felt good about my body.

We had privacy.

The atmosphere felt sexy.

I felt confident that we would have
good sex.

We had the time to have sex.

I had some alone time beforehand.

I felt desired by my partner.

I slept well the night before.

We spent lots of time kissing,
touching, or having foreplay.

Track yourself for the next few weeks and write down anything that inches you closer to Drive.

Then, consider these questions:

- What are the three most frequent dynamics that typically put you into Drive? (For example, "feeling connected throughout the day," "having some alone time," and "spending plenty of time kissing.")
- What are the three most powerful things you or your partner could do to put you into Drive more often?
- Imagine that you get offered $100,000 to write an erotic novel. What would the plot be?

The Power of Anticipation

If you're anything like Aaliyah, you're probably feeling pretty frustrated that increasing your libido isn't as easy as popping one of those tacky sex pills you always see at the gas station. So, let me try to win you back with a simple, practical way to increase your sex drive: anticipate yourself having great sex.

To explain, I have to tell you about dopamine, so let me science-geek out on you for a second. Dopamine is the hormone that helps us feel pleasure. Interestingly, research has found that the *anticipation* of pleasure increases the level of dopamine in the brain even more than *experiencing* pleasure.

And dopamine doesn't just make you feel good; it's also involved in motivation. All that anticipatory dopamine signals to the brain that an activity is worth doing. Anticipating that something will be enjoyable actually makes you feel much more motivated to do it!

Simply by imagining that you're going to have great sex, you'll feel a dramatic increase in your desire to be intimate. If you want to get in the mood, visualize yourself having great sex with your partner. The key is to be as detailed and specific as you can, so you'll need to spend some time thinking about what "good sex" means to you. (Which is a fantastically useful exercise in and of itself!) Here are some questions to think about:

- What are some of your hottest sexual memories with your partner?
- What specific sexual activities bring you the most pleasure?
- What are your favorite things to do during sex?
- What about your favorite things that your partner does?
- What does great sex feel like physically?
- What does it feel like emotionally?
- How is your life better when you have good sex?

This technique blows Aaliyah's mind. "Oh, damn, so this is making me realize that I spend the whole day anticipating being with Bryce, but I never spend any time anticipating being with Sebastian. I *used* to think about Sebastian all the time when we first started dating, but now I never do."

The previous questions will also help you transition into the second major part of your User Manual . . .

Discovering What Brings You Pleasure

If you're like most people, you have a hard time identifying what you enjoy in the bedroom. If your partner has ever whispered, "What do you want?" in your ear during sex, you likely froze up. Like Aaliyah, most of us don't like being asked this question. It feels both massive and unknowable. Like we're supposed to answer with a detailed fifteen-step plan guaranteed to make us orgasm within sixty seconds, but we also don't even know what the options are in the first place. It may be yet another way that you feel like a stranger to yourself.

But sex should be pleasurable, so I want to help you uncover what makes your toes curl!

Focus on Your Experience

In order to understand what you like, you have to be able to pay attention to your experience in the moment. Most of us are distracted during sex, and we don't end up fully registering whether or not we like something unless it's at an extreme end of the spectrum. ("Holy crap, my soul just left my body" or "That was about as enjoyable as a dental cleaning.") But there are so many more nuances that we can be open to, so let's break it down into specific categories to consider during sex. I've come up with a nifty little acronym you can use to remember them in the moment—PLEASE.

- *Position.* What position are your bodies in? Are you comfortable? Do you want to adjust your limbs in any way? If it's a sex position, are you hitting the right angles?
- *Length.* How quickly or slowly are things unfolding, and does that pace feel good to you?
- *Environment.* Do your surroundings feel sexy? Are you in a good location? Are there distractions?
- *Activity.* What specific thing are the two of you doing together? Are you enjoying that activity, or is there something different you'd rather be doing?

- *Stimulation.* Where and how is your partner touching you? Do you like being touched there? How's the pressure? What about the speed?
- *Energy.* Does the mood feel right? What kind of energy are you and your partner each bringing into the experience? What's the energy like between the two of you?

Everything Counts

Pleasure doesn't have to be elaborate. Aaliyah likes soft kisses, back scratches, and Sebastian saying "you're so good at that" when she focuses on him.

The Other Half with Xander: Look to the Past for Inspiration

Your sexual history is full of clues about what you want and like in the bedroom. Here are some places to start "investigating":

- Your early memories of or fantasies about sex. What did you think "sex" was? What felt appealing about it? Was there anything that confused you, or scared you a little about it? Was there something you couldn't stop thinking about? Even if your answers to these questions sound silly now, you might find yourself enjoying playing out some of these ideas in bed.
- Your experiences with masturbation. What do you think about when you touch yourself?
- Your favorite sexual memories, with your current or past partners. What, specifically, made sex so great in those particular moments? Have you continued to do the things that made those memories so wonderful? Or are there things you haven't done since? How could you start (re)incorporating some of those things into your sex life?

- Unsatisfying experiences. I know how tempting it can be to just want to forget about these, but they can actually be just as informative as good ones. Do you have any memories of having particularly bad sex? Or even mediocre sex? What do you think made it that way? More important, are any of the unsatisfying activities or dynamics a regular part of your current sex life?

Masturbate

I'm a huge proponent of masturbation. It's the best way to get to know your body and figure out what you like. Masturbation can help you learn how to be more present in your own skin, how to turn yourself on, and how to get yourself off. It decreases sexual shame and embarrassment, promotes body confidence, and changes your relationship with pleasure. You can literally write your User Manual with your own hand!

Most people hear the word "masturbation" and immediately think of touching their genitals. But I have a broader definition: I think of it as any sort of pleasurable touch that you give to your own body. Masturbation can be about exploring other sensitive areas of your body, too, not just what's between your legs.

Stay Open

Your likes and dislikes in the bedroom are constantly evolving, based on your experiences, new or changing relationships, and your own personal development.

Months later, after having sex with a brand-new partner, Aaliyah plops onto my couch and exclaims, "Your girl loves being tied up! Who knew?!"

You're never going to know every single detail of what makes you tick in the bedroom, and that's okay. Part of what makes sex so fun is that there's always something new to explore and learn! So, leave a few pages open at the end of your User Manual, okay?

JUST THE TIP(S):

- Before you can start talking about sex with your partner, you need to start drafting your sexual User Manual.
- Your sex drive is affected by "Me" dynamics and "We" dynamics.
- Mental desire and physical arousal function independently of each other, so it's important to know if you're a Spontaneous or Responsive sex drive type.
- It's more valuable to identify your turn-*offs* before you explore your turn-*ons*.
- What you like in the bedroom will forever be evolving, but start paying closer attention.

CHAPTER 3

SETTING YOUR RULES
OF ENGAGEMENT

THE SUBJECT LINE of the email at the top of my inbox is five fire-alarm emojis. The message inside reads: "My name is Sunil. I'm an Indian-American guy, exploring my sexuality for the first time at thirty-six years old. I grew up in a culture where homosexuality was strictly forbidden (my parents would disown me if they knew what I was up to as of late), but I've always known that I was interested in men. I've started seeing someone whom I'm quite into, and he's trying to get me to explore anal play. Maybe I'm weird, but in my fantasies, I only ever imagined penises. Hand jobs, oral sex, but never anal play. But the problem is that I like this guy a lot, I know he's very keen on anal, and I have this thing about wanting to please people...."

Safety is one of the most important foundations of a healthy sex life, yet it's rarely talked about. In order to have great sex, you have to know and enforce your boundaries—not to mention have partners who respect them. There's just no way to say yes to something unless you feel fully comfortable saying no, too. (Are you getting a hint of what my advice to Sunil is going to be?)

The challenge is that most of us don't have healthy relationships with our boundaries. Many of us, like Sunil, only have a vague sense of what our bound-

aries are. Or we feel ashamed that we want to say no to specific activities because our partner wants us to be a yes, or because we feel like we're supposed to
be "more free" or "less of a prude." (This is a message that I get a lot when I talk
about my own personal boundaries. People think that being a sex therapist, I
should be having wild sex, where anything and everything is on the table.) Our
complicated relationship with our "yesses" and "nos" makes it hard for us to understand our own User Manual, and even more difficult to speak frankly with
our partners; all the more reason to get to know our boundaries better now.

What Are We Talking About Here?

Speaking broadly, boundaries are the things we need in order to feel comfortable and safe in the world and in our relationships. They are our way of
separating our needs from others' needs and of defining what feels healthy
and unhealthy to us. Your sexual boundaries are the things you require from
yourself, your partner, and your sex life to feel safe and satisfied. They can
include words, actions, energies, specific sex acts, and so much more. I've
defined three broad categories of sexual boundaries:

- Things that don't sound sexy or pleasurable to you.
- Things that don't sound safe to you.
- Things that go against your values.

For example, let's say you've simply never been interested in trying
Doggystyle. Or you're a survivor of sexual abuse, and you know that dirty
talk freaks you out. Or you value freedom, so you wouldn't ever want to be
in a monogamous relationship. Those are all perfectly valid boundaries to
have—and to express to your partner.

Boundaries aren't always easy to pin down, though. They're constantly
shifting and evolving, and sometimes you don't know you have a limit until
after the fact. I once went into a date open to the idea of sleeping with the

guy. I'd had my fair share of casual sex before, and I was very attracted to this person. But as soon as we started kissing, things just felt off. I couldn't identify why, and the feeling wasn't that strong, so I kept going for a bit. Just a few minutes later, I surprised both of us by jumping up and telling him I needed to leave. But I knew I'd made the right call when I felt an enormous sense of relief as I drove away.

Identifying Your Boundaries

I'm going to lead you through the process of creating a list of your sexual guidelines. This will be a living, breathing document for you, one that you'll return to often to edit or add to. You'll do a similar exercise with your partner about your sexual curiosities in Conversation 5, but I want to introduce this version to you first so you can flesh out your User Manual.

Most people think of boundaries as things we want to say no to, but I like to include yes and even maybe, too. I use a red light (hard no), yellow light (maybe), and green light (excited yes) model. I like including green lights because setting your parameters doesn't have to mean focusing only on the negative or unwanted aspects of your sex life. There's a lot of joy in being able to confidently say yes to something! And I love the murkier territory of the maybe because it invites us to get curious about our boundaries and think of them in a more nuanced way. Casual sex was a maybe for me during my dating days. It depended on the person, the situation, my mood, and so many other variables.

Write down anything that comes to mind in any of the categories, no matter how small or insignificant it might seem. For example, I had a client who didn't want to be called "Mommy" in any sort of sexual context. It was just a single word, but we added it to her red lights. For things you're unsure about, try visualizing yourself doing it, in as much detail as possible, and notice what comes up for you. If you need specific ideas to get you started, skip ahead to the exercise in Conversation 5.

Red Lights: _____

_____

_____

Yellow Lights: _____

_____

_____

Green Lights: _____

_____

_____

Is It Really a Boundary?

Let me be perfectly clear: you're allowed to say no to any kind of sexual activity, for any reason. There are no gold stars awarded to those who have zero rules in the bedroom. But sometimes, the things we think of as our boundaries aren't about our safety or about values; they're reflections of ways we've been taught to be embarrassed or ashamed of sex. Sunil's story is a great example. He's entitled to say that he doesn't want anal play in the bedroom. Yet, I think it's worth his exploring where that boundary comes from. He mentioned that homosexuality isn't permissible in his family, so is it possible that cultural shame is the reason why he's not allowing himself to explore the back door? Our brains can work overtime coming up with justifications when we're in tricky territory like this; Sunil isn't the first man I've talked to who found ways to rationalize hand and blow jobs, but deemed anal play "too gay." On the other hand, Sunil also mentioned that he's a people-pleaser, and he is worried about losing his new beau if he doesn't allow for anal action. If I were working with Sunil, I would want to ensure that he feels comfortable saying no to his new partner. See how boundaries can quickly get complicated?

Here's another example. Maybe you're a vulva owner who has never wanted to let your partner go down on you because you grew up hearing too many jokes about tuna fish and roast-beef curtains. That's not about oral sex not feeling safe to you, nor does it go against your values. That's about being taught to be ashamed of your body. It's an external discomfort, not an internal one.

It's also important to note the difference between boundaries and preferences. I personally don't love vibrators. For me, the sensation feels like too much, too fast, and I don't find my toy-induced orgasms particularly pleasurable or satisfying. But that doesn't inherently mean I have a boundary against using toys in the bedroom.

Take this moment to get curious about your boundaries. Ask yourself these questions about each of your red lights:

"Are there any safety- or value-based reasons why I've said no to this?" (If you can identify just one dynamic, you can skip the remainder of these questions.)

"Why might I be having a reaction to this activity?"

"Is it serving me to say no to this?"

"Do I want to keep this boundary?"

The goal here is not to eliminate all your boundaries but rather to feel stronger about them. Giving yourself this permission to examine your boundaries on an ongoing basis will be so powerful for you, and it's going to set you up to have more meaningful conversations with your partner, too.

Navigating Trauma

Maria couldn't believe her luck when Jax agreed to go to prom with her. She was a lowly sophomore, with a small group of friends who were on the "B-list" of their high school's social order. Jax was a senior, wealthy, popular, and headed off to the well-renowned state school on a soccer scholarship. Maria couldn't imagine a universe where Jax would have invited her to the prom, but his equally rich and good-looking girlfriend, Laurel, had caught him cheating the week before, leaving Jax with no date and no good backup options. Maria had been tutoring Jax in Spanish for the whole year, so they had formed a transactional connection. When Jax had showed up at their last session glumly complaining that he'd have to go to prom alone like a loser, Maria shocked herself by blurting out, "I'll go with you!"

Prom was a dream. Jax and his friends mostly ignored her, but she was thrilled just to be there—and to be seen with them. Jax snuck her a few drinks from his smuggled flasks, and even let her tag along to a private after-party.

But just a few hours later, Maria's world was shattered when Jax forced himself on her.

———

Sexual abuse is frighteningly common. One in five women and one in four-teen men experience attempted or completed rape in their lifetime. Nearly half of all women will experience some form of sexual violence in their lifetime.[1] For transgender and nonbinary people, those numbers can be even higher.[2] If you're a part of that group, first of all, I just want to say that I'm so deeply sorry. You've gone through something that no human being should ever have to endure. The actual experience of being abused is horrible enough, but unfortunately abuse can have lasting impacts on your sex life. You didn't and don't deserve any of this, and I'm sorry you have to shoulder that burden.

That being said, I want to assure you that you can still have a healthy and happy sex life after experiencing abuse. I highly recommend getting personal therapy to help you process the effects of the abuse and reconnect with your body and your sexuality. This section is not meant to be a replace-ment for psychotherapy, but since abuse is so prevalent, I do want to use Maria's story to highlight some of the ways that abuse can impact your sex life in the hopes that, at the very least, you feel less alone.

Maria became my client ten years after she was assaulted. She's engaged to Jesse, a kind, sensitive, and patient man. Maria told Jesse about the abuse, and they cried together. He told her he would never, ever hurt her like that, and she believed him. But neither of them understands why it has been so challenging to have a great sex life together. Like many survivors, Maria downplays and minimizes her abuse. "It was ages ago," she says, "and I know so many women had it worse than I did. I'm over it, so I don't get why Jesse and I are struggling."

The first issue that we discuss is Maria's avoidance of physical intimacy. Like so many sexual abuse survivors, Maria isn't particularly interested in sex. I explain to her that low libido can be a defense mechanism. Her first experience with sex was traumatic, so her body has learned that sex is unsafe, undesired, and painful. Even though her brain understands that Jesse is not Jax, her body has shut down her sex drive in an attempt to protect her from being hurt again.

Maria's sexual history between Jax and Jesse makes things feel more complicated for her. She had a number of casual sex encounters, often with partners who showed her very little respect, and she made some risky decisions that she now feels ashamed of. She asks, "Why did I seek out so much sex with men who didn't care about me at all, but I don't want it with a man who loves me and treats me right?" Even the beginning of Maria and Jesse's relationship now feels baffling. Maria seemed wild and uninhibited in the first few months, and they had sex often. It wasn't until things got serious between them that she started retreating, leaving Jesse wondering where his sex kitten girlfriend had disappeared to.

When we get into the deepest part of the work, Maria confesses that she blames herself for the rape. I tell her that no one ever deserves to be assaulted, but she presents me with two pieces of "evidence": her post-rape sexual decision-making, and the fact that she got wet during the attack.

This is one of the most confusing and painful side effects of sexual abuse, so I want to make sure I explain it carefully. In the last chapter, I told you that there's a difference between mental desire (wanting sex) and physical arousal (your body preparing for sex). There's a term for when your brain and your body aren't on the same page: "nonconcordance." One of the most extreme examples of nonconcordance can happen during abuse. Even though every fiber of your being doesn't *want* the experience of being assaulted, your body may still *respond*. Vulva owners can get wet. Penis owners can get hard. People of all genders can even orgasm. I want to be extremely clear: having a nonconcordant reaction does not mean that your body "wanted" to have sex. It just means that it was responding to stimuli. Think about eating a lemon or a pickle. Your mouth is naturally going to start to produce saliva. You can try really hard to keep your mouth dry, but you're just not going to be able to. Our bodies simply respond to stimuli.

Most sexual abuse survivors never learn about nonconcordance, so it leads to a distrustful relationship with their bodies. Like Maria, you might blame yourself for your assault. Or you may feel like your body betrayed you. If you had a physical reaction to your trauma, I want you to understand that this is common, and it in no way means that you wanted or enjoyed the abuse. Your body is not your enemy.

Maria and Jesse do have sex occasionally, when Maria gets overwhelmed by her guilt about how long it's been since the last time they had sex. She tells Jesse, "You can do your thing." He feels torn because he wants her to be present and excited about physical intimacy, but he's also so desperate to connect with her that he's sometimes willing to settle for scraps.

When they have sex, Maria exhibits one of the classic signs of sexual abuse: dissociation. This occurs when you experience a disconnection between your brain and your body, as if they were operating independently of each other. All of us experience dissociation in mild forms in everyday life. Have you ever had the experience of pulling into your driveway, but having no recollection of driving home? Your body was able to follow your usual route, even though your brain was somewhere else entirely in the moment.

When I explain dissociation to Maria, she realizes that she dissociated during the rape itself. She describes her spirit leaving her body. "It was like I was floating up in the air, looking down at myself being assaulted." This brings up shame for her, so I gently tell her that dissociation is an amazing defense mechanism. "Your spirit knew that it was unsafe to be in your body during the abuse, so it got the hell out of there. If you had been mentally and emotionally present, it would only serve to make the experience that much more painful. You were forced to be there physically, but at least your spirit got out of there and spared you some amount of pain."

Unfortunately, dissociation can persist long after the abuse is over. Your brain gets the message that it's not safe to be in your body during sex, so it just keeps taking off whenever it looks like things might be headed in that direction. You may find it really hard to be present during sex, even if you're with a trusted partner. Maria realizes that she's almost always dissociating during sex. Jesse tells me he notices it, too.

Even nonsexual physical intimacy can feel challenging for Maria and Jesse. Like many survivors, Maria is jumpy about physical contact. Jesse tells me, "It feels like she's always on guard and suspicious of me, even when I'm just trying to give her a hug." It pains him when he reaches out to touch her and feels her tense up. I explain to them both that Maria's brain rationally understands that she's not being abused anymore, but her body is still holding on to the trauma. Her body is hypervigilant, constantly on the lookout for danger. I help Maria identify the specific words, actions, sounds, gestures, and even smells that can send her into a heightened state of agitation, and we come up with a game plan for avoiding, minimizing, or navigating her hypervigilance. As we start making progress, she tells me, "I didn't realize how much energy I've been spending staying on the alert all the time. I'm exhausted."

As I said before, this chapter is not meant to serve as a replacement for therapy. You deserve to have a safe container and a trusted guide for your healing process. But I hope that hearing Maria's story helps you understand some of the experiences or reactions you may have had since the abuse, and that encourages you to seek support. (If you're looking for further resources, we offer a free course for survivors of sexual assault at vmtherapy .com/book.)

The Other Half with Xander:
Being a Good Partner to Someone Who Has Experienced Abuse

If you're not a survivor yourself, you'll never be able to *fully* understand what your partner is going through. It's normal to feel confused or lost about how to best support them, so here are some tips:

- Let your partner know you're open to hearing their story. "Open" is the key word here: make yourself available to listen, but don't pressure them into sharing immediately or more than they're comfortable with.
- Educate yourself about the impacts of sexual abuse. Your being informed beforehand will make you a better partner and listener.
- Get to know your partner's boundaries and treat them with the utmost care and respect. You can even work on identifying and discussing your own boundaries, too, so your partner doesn't need to feel like they're the only one with "rules."
- Your partner will likely continue to be reminded of their abuse from time to time. You can be an ongoing source of support by continuing to listen, letting them feel their feelings, reiterating that you're on their team, and checking in to see if they need anything from you.
- Keep telling your partner that you love, value, and respect them. It's easy for survivors to feel like "damaged goods."
- Encourage your partner to get as much support as they can, whether that's psychotherapy, sex therapy, support groups, crisis lines, or talking to trusted loved ones. Offer to be a part of their healing process, in whatever way feels good to them. Just remember that it's ultimately up to them to make the decisions about how they recover and heal.

Unpacking Your Sexual Baggage

When you start having the Sex Talks with your partner, it's very likely that your limiting beliefs about sex are going to get in your way. For example, it would be hard to even ask your partner to read this book with you if you think sex is something you're not supposed to talk about openly. (Just like my parents struggled to have "the talk" with me in our minivan.) In order to maximize your chances of having successful conversations later, let's start tackling your beliefs together.

I'm going to walk you through an exercise I developed called the Take This Back Technique. It's a simple process, and while not a substitute for personal therapy, it can be a great way to start dismantling your blockages.

Make a list of any negative, limiting, or unwanted beliefs you have about sex. As you write each one down, start with the phrase, "There's a part of me that believes . . ." For example, "There's a part of me that thinks that my body is unworthy of attention" or "There's a part of me that believes that asking for what I want will be insulting to my partner." No matter how strong your blockages may seem, you don't feel them in every fiber of your being. I like phrasing beliefs in this way because it makes them more manageable to work with. It's similar to the inner-critic exercise I shared in the last chapter. Our goal is to help you realize that you are not your blockages.

There's part of me that believes:

_____

_____

_____

There's part of me that thinks:

_____

_____

_____

There's part of me that feels:

_____

_____

_____

There's part of me that fears:

_____

_____

_____

Take the time to identify where each of these beliefs originated. Did you first hear it from your parents? Did your religion teach you this? Your culture? Your friends at school?

I believe these ideas came from:

_____

_____

_____

This step helps you realize that all the BS we've been taught to believe about sex is external. None of us was born being inherently ashamed of or embarrassed about sex!

Religion is a common source of sexual blockages, since many religious teachings about sex are shame filled, strict, avoidant, and oftentimes contradictory. Francesca once shared with me: "My religion told me that I couldn't have sex until I was married, and that I would be 'impure' and 'undesirable' if I didn't wait. Then the instant I became a wife, I became responsible for pleasing my husband 24/7. But I can't just flip a switch. It's hard to develop a healthy relationship with sex if you've been told your entire life that it's sinful and the root of all evil."

Working with one blockage at a time, visualize whoever it was that taught it to you, and imagine yourself handing that baggage back to them. Say to the person or entity that you're handing it over to: "I don't want this anymore. It's not mine, and it's not serving me. I'd like you to take this back." Your blockages aren't going to disappear the instant you imagine handing them over (I don't want to make this process seem as simple as "flipping a switch"), but doing this visualization will help you start to regain your sense of agency. And of course, therapy can be extremely beneficial in helping you untangle deeper beliefs.

Creating Your Own Terms

To wrap this chapter up, start by making a list of your goals for your sex life. It's easy to feel overwhelmed by all the blockages and limiting beliefs we're all burdened with, and to forget that there are also a lot of amazing, positive things to work toward! Having a healthy relationship with your sexuality isn't just about overcoming hurdles; it's also about joyfully defining and claiming your own goals. For example, maybe you want to initiate sex with confidence, learn how to orgasm, or bring your true self into the bedroom. The more specific and detailed you can get with your goals, the better! You can even work from your blockages: Examine each limiting thought and write down what you *want* to believe instead.

I encourage you to let your partner in on your process. The wild thing about limiting beliefs is that they're often shared. Most of us tend to feel like we're being crushed by the weight of our baggage all by our lonesome, but the odds are that your partner has much of the same baggage. (A matching set of luggage, you might say!) There's an opportunity to bond about the crap you're both carrying. Plus, these types of beliefs tend to lose their power over us once we bring them out into the light of day.

Your Sexual Goals

_____

_____

_____

_____

_____

_____

_____

Now that you've worked out your boundaries, your beliefs, and your goals, you're in control of your own sex life. You get to decide how you think and feel about sex, what you do, and who you choose to share yourself with.

JUST THE TIP(S):

- You're allowed to have boundaries against things that don't sound sexy or safe to you, or that go against your values. But be on the lookout for boundaries that are the result of internalized shame rather than authentic guidelines.
- Sexual abuse can have lasting impacts, including low sex drive, hypervigilance, unsafe decision-making, bad body image, and dissociation, but it is possible to create a healthy sex life after assault.
- We all have negative, limited, and unwanted beliefs about sex, and it's our responsibility to work on unpacking them individually.
- Coming up with specific and detailed goals for your sex life is one of the best ways to regain control and find joy.

CHAPTER 4

BUILDING THE FOUNDATION FOR YOUR SEX TALKS

IN THE NEXT section, you're going to get started with your Sex Talks. These conversations are obviously going to require open, honest communication. Unfortunately, most of us are kinda sucky at the whole talking thing. So, let's set some basic ground rules. Nine of them, to be specific. Think of this as your crash course in communication.

The Golden Rules of the Five Sex Talks

1: NAME YOUR INTENTIONS

People get pretty damned nervous about communication, especially when it involves sex. Those nerves lead us to rehearse conversations in our head, imagining dozens of horrible scenarios of how they can go wrong. But here's what you need to remind yourself: you have good intentions and positive goals driving your desire to communicate. It's not like you picked up this book thinking, *I hope Vanessa teaches me the best ways to destroy my partner's confidence and ruin our relationship.* Remind yourself of your positive intentions often, especially before approaching your partner. Take a deep breath and tell yourself, "I'm initiating this conversation because I love my partner and I know we're capable of a smoking-hot sex life." Giving yourself this pep talk can soothe your anxiety and help you go into the conversation feeling stronger.

It can also be helpful to set intentions with your partner before starting a conversation. Xander and I start any serious chat by asking each other, "What's your intention in having this conversation?" That way, you're setting yourselves up for success right from the beginning. Even if things wind up feeling weird or uncomfortable, there's an understanding that you're working together toward a more intimate relationship. Keep in mind that your intentions don't need to be complicated. They can be as simple as "We want to have a calm and loving conversation."

2: SEE YOURSELVES AS A TEAM

One of the best things you can do for your relationship is think of you and your partner as teammates, working together against whatever is getting in the way of having the sex life of your wildest dreams. No one partner is the problem child. You are two individuals who brought history, complications, and ever-evolving needs to your relationship, and your task is to spread all of it out in front of you and say, "Okay, how do we make sense of this together?" As you're reading through the rest of this book, take a "What's mine is yours, and what's yours is mine" kind of approach to your challenges, and think about how your puzzle pieces fit together.

Give your teammate the benefit of the doubt during your Sex Talks. If things start to get heated, it can be easy to feel like your partner is purposefully trying to hurt or upset you. And they're probably going to be thinking the exact same thing about you! Challenge yourself to think about the good intentions that your partner has in every situation. (That's why reminding each other of your intentions right before a conversation can be so powerful.) Ask yourself, "What positive feeling does my partner want from their words or actions—even if they're going about things in an unskillful manner?"

3: START SOFTLY

Research has found that the way you start a conversation predicts how it will end. In fact, relationship expert John Gottman is famous for being able to predict the likelihood of a couple's divorce by observing just the first three minutes of a conflict discussion.[1] The way that you start conversations is *that* important!

When it comes to having your Sex Talks, make sure the conditions are right. Don't try to talk to your partner when they're cooking dinner, when they need to leave in ten minutes to get to a doctor's appointment, or when they're obviously stressed about a looming work deadline. Check in with yourself, too. There's a helpful acronym that you can use here: HALT. If you feel Hungry, Angry, Lonely, or Tired, take a moment to address those feelings before talking to your partner. Only initiate conversations when you both have the space and energy to properly have them. For instance, I have a bad habit of ambushing Xander with complaints when we're already swamped. We'll be running out the door to take the pugs to the vet, and I'll harp on him for leaving all his beard trimmings in the sink. It's essentially setting him up for failure, since there's no way he can address or even fully listen to my request, and it leaves both of us feeling combative. (Note to self: stop doing this.)

Another way to start softly is to initiate any big conversations by labeling your baggage. Acknowledge the challenges you or your partner have faced or are currently facing when it comes to having a healthy relationship with intimacy. For example, "I know we were both raised Catholic, and are still carrying a lot of shame about sex." This reminds you both that your difficulties aren't your fault, that there are understandable reasons why you're struggling, and that you're a team.

Here's a funny trick you can use to soften your delivery. Imagine that you're talking to a friend instead of your partner. Most of us listen to our friends more closely, and we have lower expectations and more patience for them. We tend to give them the benefit of the doubt, and we don't get as triggered by what they say or do. Imagine one of your best friends in front of you when you're talking to your partner, and watch your communication transform. This is a fun hack to play with, and it's surprisingly effective in the moment!

Here are a few other ways to start softly:

- Keep your tone calm and even.
- Be aware of your facial expressions and body language, and try to convey relaxation.
- If you're open to it, hold hands or touch while you talk. A little bit of physical contact reminds you of your love for each other.
- Make sure your first few sentences are particularly kind and open.

4: USE "I" LANGUAGE

You've probably heard this one before; it's an oldie but a goodie. Instead of saying "You did this" or "You did that," talk about your personal reactions and experiences using "I," "me," and "my." So instead of, "You never want to spend time with me," you say, "I've been feeling lonely lately, and I've been wanting to feel more connected to you." If you're feeling stuck, here's an easy framework to use: "I feel X, and I need Y." Notice how that worked in the prior example—I'm feeling *lonely* and I need more *connection*.

Using "I" language cuts defensiveness off at the pass. If you tell your partner, "You did this," it's going to feel like an attack to them, and it's likely to trigger an argumentative response like "No, I didn't!" But if you talk about your own experience, it's less likely to inflame that defensiveness.

This also helps you identify the feelings that are coming up for you. Your feelings are what need tending to when you're upset, not the actual details of what happened. I'll give you a great example: If you say, "You haven't initiated sex in months," your partner is going to respond with something like, "Yes I have! I did three weeks ago." Then the conversation turns into a debate about exactly how many weeks it's been since they initiated. "No, it's been months." "No, the last time was before Rudy's birthday party and that was *this* month."

But what about your *feelings* about initiation? Are you feeling sad? Lonely? Resentful? All those emotions get lost. And the worst part of it all? You're never, ever going to agree about the logistics. You're going to be convinced about your timeline, your partner is going to be convinced about their timeline, and those two things are never going to match up. It's the feelings that matter, and so using "I" language will help you access that deeper layer.

5: GO SLOW

This golden rule has two meanings: go at a slow speed, and tackle things one at a time!

Most of us tend to speed up when we're nervous or upset. Your partner senses you starting to get more intense, and they get more intense in response. Before you know it, you're having a conversation at breakneck pace. But going fast creates a lot of problems:

- You're much more likely to interpret your partner's words as negative, even if they're not.
- You're much less likely to listen fully.
- You're much less likely to express yourself properly. When you're going too fast, you end up stumbling over your own thoughts and words.

So, slow the eff down! Sometimes I even tell my clients, "Have a conversation at fifty percent of your usual speed." Another practical trick is to make yourself take a deep breath before every sentence you speak. This naturally slows you down and helps you relax.

6: WHAT TO ALWAYS DO TO NEVER FIGHT

Just kidding! "Always" and "never" are two of the least helpful words for couples. Let's just get one thing out of the way first: it's extremely rare in life that something *always* happens or *never* happens. It's just not accurate language. Plus, these two little words will immediately put your partner on the defensive and make them feel trapped. If they "always" or "never" do something, then you're essentially saying they're incapable of doing anything different.

These words also set the bar pathetically low for improvement. Let's say you tell your partner, "You never give me compliments." All your partner needs to do is give you one compliment to prove you wrong. Can't you just picture them smarmily saying, "See, I told you!" And it will put the two of you right back into that argument about logistics. So, do yourselves a favor and eliminate those two words from your vocabulary.

7: MAKE SPACE FOR NEW BEHAVIORS

You want your partner to change? Then you need to make the space for them to actually change! Rashida dragged her husband, Anthony, into a couples session because she wanted him to be more aggressive and dominant in the bedroom. "But he'll never do it," she said. "He's too shy." Anthony was seated right beside her on the sofa, staring intently at his feet. Want to hear the shocker of the century? He didn't change a thing. Rashida sabotaged any possibility of getting her own wish.

8: CLOSE YOUR MOUTH AND OPEN YOUR EARS

You know you have to let your partner speak, too, right? Your tasks as a listener are to try your best to understand your partner and to help them feel seen. Kick off your own shoes for a minute, and try to put on your partner's. Give them your full and undivided attention (no multitasking!). Make eye contact. Turn your body toward theirs.

There's a little trick that you'll learn in any Psychology 101 class: active listening. After your partner has finished talking, try to summarize what they just said, in your own words. Start with, "So, what I'm hearing is . . ." or "What that sounded like to me is . . ." Ask them if you've correctly captured it. If your partner says, "Not exactly," ask them to clarify what they originally meant. This makes it clear to your partner that it's important to you to truly understand what they're trying to say, and it will cut off misunderstandings before they snowball into huge fights. I'll give you a heads-up that this technique will feel super clunky at first, but it's so worth it.

9: BE COMPASSIONATE

You're going to see me repeat this over and over again: we all have our baggage when it comes to sex. You have your stuff, your partner has their stuff, Xander and I have our own stuff. If your partner is struggling, try to be empathetic and recognize that they're dealing with their own internal wounds about sex. The best way to get a derailed conversation back on the tracks is to remind yourselves that you're both doing the best you can. It will get easier with practice, I promise!

The Other Half with Xander: Communication Hacks

Here are a few communication tricks that have made huge impacts on my life:

Don't ask questions that aren't questions

Earlier in our relationship, Vanessa and I often struggled to ask for what we really wanted, and we'd find ourselves hiding our needs and requests in more logistical questions. If I was working late and Vanessa was feeling lonely, she might ask me, "Are you almost done with that?" or "Are you going to be home soon?" Thinking that I was answering her simple question, I might respond with something straightforward like, "No, I have to spend a couple more hours finishing this project." But Vanessa would come away with hurt feelings, because what she really intended to ask was, "I miss you; can you spend some time with me?"

We've since learned that hiding requests in questions only serves to set your partner up for failure. They think they're just supposed to answer the objective question, not address the unspoken emotional need beneath it. Instead, take a second to think about what need or request you actually have, and ask for it outright. In Vanessa's and my example above, she could have told me she was feeling lonely, and while I may have still explained that I had too much work to come home immediately, I would have at least had a chance to express how much I missed her, too, and my desire to spend time with her!

Don't anticipate what your partner is going to say

I'm a verbal processer and a slower talker, and Vanessa will frequently jump to conclusions about what she thinks I'm going to say. Then she'll start responding to me based on the scenario she's concocted in her mind. I can't tell you how many times I've had to tell her, "Babe, that's not even what I was about to say." This dynamic can be harmless in everyday chitchat, but in any sort of serious conversation, having your partner interrupt and make assumptions can quickly turn it into a full-blown fight.

Don't plan your response in your head as your partner is talking

I know from experience just how tempting it is to think about what to say next or how to defend yourself when your partner is talking. Especially if you think you have a pretty good idea of what they're about to say! But instead, remind yourself that you aren't actually a mind reader and practice your active listening so you can *really* try to understand what your partner is saying or how they're feeling. When you're truly listening and not planning your response, you probably won't be able to start responding to your partner the millisecond they stop talking. And that's okay! Just tell your partner you're taking a couple of seconds to collect your thoughts.

How the Next Section Works

It's time to move into the heart of *Sex Talks*: the five crucial conversations that every couple needs to have about their sex life. This section is divided into chapters based on the most common challenges couples come across. We'll cover:

1. Acknowledgment, aka, "Sex Is a Thing and We Have It"
2. Connection, aka, "What Do We Need to Feel Close to Each Other?"
3. Desire, aka, "What Do We Each Need to Get Turned On?"
4. Pleasure, aka, "What Do We Each Need to Feel Good?"
5. Exploration, aka, "What Should We Try Next?"

The goal is for you and your partner to have all five conversations, but you'll probably discover that there's one specific area that causes the most tension in your relationship. For example, Xander and I struggle the most with Connection. When we're not spending quality time together or having meaningful conversations, it throws off our energy in the bedroom, too. If you're curious about identifying your relationship's weak point, there's a quiz on page 237, at the end of the book. That being said, my recommendation is to go through the conversations in the order they're presented.

I've included a section at the end of each chapter called "Navigating Common Pitfalls." I've tested all these communication techniques on thousands of clients, so I've been able to identify the unique ways that couples can get tripped up, and I've armed you with tips to prepare yourselves in advance.

The Three Promises

To truly get the most out of this journey, I want you to make three promises to yourself and to your partner:

> "I promise to give this my best, even when I feel scared, anxious, self-conscious, or embarrassed."

"I promise to give you the benefit of the doubt that you're trying your best, too, even if your words or actions sometimes hurt me."

"I promise to remind myself that a hot and healthy sex life is a goal worth working toward, and that we're on the same team in trying to get there."

Ready? Let's do this!

Part Two

THE FIVE
SEX TALKS

CHAPTER 5

THE FIRST CONVERSATION:
Acknowledgment

aka, "Sex Is a Thing and We Have It"

THERE WAS A single finger in my butt.

And I wasn't quite sure how I felt about it.

I'd felt his hand starting to snake back around there. I experienced that moment that many vulva owners are familiar with when there's a body part between our legs: "Okay, here we go. . . . Wait a second . . . you're passing the intended target. . . . Oh no, go back before it's too late! . . . Hold up, *is this intentional?!*"

It was my first foray into anal play, and to be perfectly honest, it felt pretty good. But it was also my first time hooking up with this new guy, and I wasn't sure I felt ready to explore the great unknown of my butthole with him.

And yet, I didn't say anything. I felt ashamed even acknowledging that I had a butthole in the first place, since all things anal are still pretty taboo. I didn't want to interrupt the flow with, "Excuse me, sir; could you take your finger out of my anus so we can have a quick chat about it first?" I didn't want my partner to think I was being a prude, or that I was insulting his sexual prowess. I wasn't sure what I would say even if I *did* feel comfortable opening my mouth. "Hey, bud, I'm kinda into this, but also kinda wish you had given me a heads-up before. But, uh, don't stop?"

It struck me in that moment how odd it is that it's so rare to talk about sex. Even with the people with whom we're *having* sex.

The man in question and I didn't even talk about this event until many years later, when I was writing this very book.

"Are you talking about *me?*" Xander asked, as he perused an early draft of this chapter. There was genuine confusion in his voice.

"Duh!" I responded.

"I have no recollection of putting my finger in your butt," he said, slowly and thoughtfully. I could see him replaying our sexual history in his head, examining it for anal clues.

"You absolutely did," I insisted.

"Weird," he responded. "I guess I did."

I couldn't help but burst into laughter. "How did we not talk about this for *fourteen years?*"

Dear reader, this complete and utter lack of communication is *not* what I want you to imitate. Instead, here's an example of what Xander's and my new and improved sexual communication looks like:

"You know what I started randomly thinking about today?" I asked Xander. "Our anniversary lunch in South Africa."

To anyone else, this conversation would have seemed innocent. But Xander shot me a little side eye and a smirk, because he knew the full story. It was 2019, and we were celebrating our eight-year wedding anniversary by taking an epic trip to South Africa. We were on safari on the big day, and the lodge we were staying at arranged for us to have a private lunch in an actual tree fort overlooking an elephant watering hole. It was already the most over-the-top anniversary celebration we'd ever had, but after finishing our lunch, we started glancing over at the lounging area in the tree house.

There was a whole cushion setup with pillows and blankets. I mean, they were just asking for people to have sex there, right? So, we did what seemed logical, and had sex in the wildest place we've ever done it—in a tree fort, in the middle of the African bush, to the soundtrack of elephants trumpeting.

This is how I recommend getting started talking about sex. Not by replicating our African safari experience (though I highly recommend that, too!), but by referencing one of the most fun memories the two of you share about your sex life. Isn't that one of the best parts of being in a relationship—having inside jokes and secrets? So, why not use them to your advantage to get the conversation going?

———

You may have been imagining that I'd kick off this chapter by telling you to confess your wildest fantasies or your biggest sexual secrets. But for so many couples, talking about sex has to start with even *acknowledging* that sex exists and that you're having it. Most of us don't talk about it very often—or at all—even with the person who regularly sees us naked. It's the big, sexy elephant (ha!) lurking in the corner of our bedrooms.

Olivia, a member of our Instagram community, told us, "My husband refuses to talk about sex because he doesn't believe it's normal for couples to have to talk about it. He has a hard time accepting that sex takes work in a long-term relationship, and it doesn't happen spontaneously. When I bring it up, he responds as if it's a confrontation, or we're in an argument."

Or take Jenny and Robert, a couple in their twenties. Their sex life has sputtered down to once a month when they're both drunk after date night. Jenny wants to talk about it, but every time she starts tiptoeing into the conversation, Robert immediately shuts down, and they'll wind up having even less sex for the next few months. In an email to me, Jenny wrote, "How did we get to a point where we literally can't even say the word 'sex'? It's instant pressure for him."

But sex is an incredibly intimate act, and not even acknowledging its existence can feel jarring. Have you ever walked into a room and had someone refuse to recognize your presence? Acknowledgment seems like a simple thing, but not having it can be exquisitely painful. Could you imagine doing this with any other aspect of your relationship? What would it look like if you and your partner never, ever talked about your kids or your finances?

Plus, if you're not openly talking about sex, minor misunderstandings can turn into major problems. Alina, a woman in our Instagram community, reached out to us to share her experience with period sex after we talked about it in our Stories. Her husband refused to be intimate with her during that time of her cycle. She told us, "I thought he was grossed out, and that was making me feel ashamed of my body. I felt undesired and undesirable, and was resentful of him for rejecting me." But our story emboldened her, and she decided to directly ask him why he didn't want to have period sex. He told her, "When I see blood, it makes me worry that I'm hurting you." He didn't think her body was gross; he was afraid he was causing her harm.

It's likely that the Acknowledgment conversation is going to be the necessary starting point for your Sex Talks adventure, which is why I've placed this conversation first. But if you're still unsure about whether or not you should start here, my question to you is this: Have you ever had a relaxed and productive conversation about sex with your partner?

This Acknowledgment conversation is all about putting the good stuff first. Not only is this easier and a whole lot more fun, it's also more effective. We're going to focus on being light, positive, and non-goal-oriented. We're not going to criticize or complain. We're not going to try to solve any problems. We're just going to get *comfortable*. This will help you and your partner build a solid foundation of sexual communication and trust.

From there, we'll get you to the point where you can suggest trying a sex position as easily as you can suggest ordering Mexican for dinner. ("You know what sounds great tonight? Some Reverse Cowgirl!") Once you get more comfortable talking about sex in a positive or even neutral way, you'll feel more confident bringing up the trickier stuff in later chapters.

"I've never even said these words out loud!"

The second she sits down on my sofa, Rowena's eyes start darting around the room, as if she's already plotting a quick escape.

"I can't believe I'm here," she says, her voice barely above a whisper. I know from her initial email that Rowena wants to talk about her orgasm. She's never had one, but she's been faking them with her husband of three years, Hakeem.

"What does it feel like to be here?" I ask her. When a client is as nervous as Rowena, you have to let them set the pace of a session. She starts crying immediately.

"I'm so broken," she says as tears slowly make their way down her cheeks. "Please tell me how to fix myself so I can be good for my husband. I don't want him to find out my secret."

I don't think Rowena is damaged goods, so I'm not going to help her furtively "fix" herself. Instead, I'm going to teach her how to talk about her pleasure with Hakeem. But I know that for Rowena—as is the case with most of my clients—we have to start with helping her get comfortable talking about sex on her own, before she can even imagine talking to Hakeem. It's not because she's broken or has to keep hiding her truth from him; she simply needs to build up her confidence.

At the end of our session, I lead her through an exercise to start laying that foundation. I ask her to pick one word that she has a hard time saying. She raises her eyebrows at me and says, "Sex! Even that word feels so scary. We never say it in my culture." I ask her to say "sex" out loud, over and over, telling her that repetition is one of the most powerful confidence-building tools. Eventually, she starts laughing. "Okay, it's feeling easier now," she tells me. I guide her over to a mirror and ask her to look at herself as she says the word. (I tell her that making eye contact with herself will mimic some of the vulnerability she might feel when she eventually talks to Hakeem.) After a dozen repetitions, she takes a deep breath. We come up with a list of other words that make her feel uncomfortable, and I send her home with instructions to repeat the steps on her own.

If you're feeling too nervous to talk to your partner yet, I encourage you to try this exercise yourself. While you're doing it, spend some time getting a sense of the words that feel best for you. Language is so personal, and it's okay for you to have your preferences. For example, one vulva-owning member of our Instagram community told me, "I despise the word 'pussy.' I get that it feels like a liberating word to some, but it makes my skin crawl. For a while I was trying to force myself to use it, as if getting comfortable with that word was a sign that I was 'sexually progressive.' But I learned from you that it's okay for me to choose my own words."

Seeing Your Partner with Fresh Eyes

Before we get to the full Acknowledgment conversation, there's one preparation step I want you to take: start giving your partner compliments. When was the last time you gave your partner a specific and positive piece of feedback? My guess is that it's been too long, so let's fix that with a structured game plan.

Kick off the compliments by telling your partner how attracted you are to them. Keep your comments light, playful, and flirty. Even if your partner has a hard time taking a compliment, it's still going to register that you're making a new effort. It's fine if your partner doesn't reciprocate the compliments for now; the point is just to open the conversational door. Give your partner a compliment a day for one week. Here are some examples you can use for inspiration:

"Look at those arm muscles! Come wrap them around me."

"Wow, you're beautiful. I can't take my eyes off you."

"Damn, you're looking good today."

"That shirt is so flattering on you. It brings out the color of your eyes."

"Did you know I'm still as attracted to you as I was the day we met?"

If you're having a hard time coming up with compliments, get creative and look for the little things. Attraction is all about paying attention. Does your partner have nice hands? A gentle smile? Cute dimples right above their butt? It's normal for attraction to fade in a relationship—especially if things have been tense lately—but it will naturally increase as you work your way through this book. For now, actively look for the things you appreciate.

Once you've gotten more comfortable with giving compliments, it's time to officially acknowledge your sex life. I'm going to give you two Choose Your Own Adventure paths for proceeding, based on whether you're the one initiating the conversation or if you and your partner are reading this book together. If you're reading this book together, skip ahead to page 74.

Let's Do This

Getting Started on Your Own

Approach your partner when they're in a good mood, the vibe is calm, and you're outside the bedroom. Here are my two favorite openers:

OPTION 1: THE AFRICAN SAFARI METHOD

"You know what I started randomly thinking about today?" Then a quick sentence or two about your favorite sexual memory with your partner.

OPTION 2: THE HOT POTATO METHOD

If you feel nervous starting with your own memory, you can put the responsibility on your partner's shoulders with this slight tweak: "What's your favorite sexual memory with me?" If you're worried about catching your partner off-guard with the question, you can soften the approach by saying something like "I know this isn't something we usually talk about, but I had a funny question pop into my head today, and I wanted to ask you. What's your favorite sexual memory with me?" Make sure you have your own answer ready to share with your partner, too.

When I see a new couple in my practice, one of the first things I say is: "Tell me about the best sex you've had together." Even if the couple is in a tough spot, reminiscing about their favorite intimate moments almost always lightens the energy in the room. They often give each other knowing glances or little giggles, and I can see the question "Are we *really* going to tell her about that?" pass between them. This prompt helps couples feel hopeful because they're reminded that they have it in them to be passionate and playful.

After you've both shared a fun memory, change the subject and talk about something else. If your partner presses you about why you brought it up, say something light like, "It just popped into my head, that's all!"

TRY IT DIGITALLY

If the idea of talking about sex face-to-face is making your palms sweat, send one of the conversation openers to your partner via email or text instead. I want you to get to the point where you feel comfortable with face-to-face conversations, but texting can be a great baby step for building your confidence and courage.

OFFER PRAISE

A day or two after that first conversation, loop back around and let your partner know that you enjoyed talking about sex with them. Make sure to give them lots of praise. Say something like, "I realize I asked you a pretty out-of-the-blue question about our sex life the other day, but I liked talking to you about it! It made me feel close to you. Thanks for being willing to have that conversation with me." You're starting to create a link between emotional and physical intimacy, and you're showing your partner that communication plays a big role in helping you feel close.

If that initial conversation felt tough for one or both of you, that's okay! Add something like, "I want us to both feel comfortable talking about sex, but, wow, it's really hard, isn't it? I'm proud that we're both willing to keep trying even though it's challenging."

KEEP THE COMPLIMENTS GOING (AND THE PRESSURE LOW)

Once you've had one good (or even neutral) chat about your sexy times together, you may be tempted to jump into all the other stuff you've been wanting to tell your partner. Like, "Okay, I told him he has a cute butt. Now it's time for him to hear how annoying it is that he comes so quickly."

Don't go there just yet! If sex isn't a regular topic of conversation in your relationship, your partner might still be a little suspicious, waiting for the other shoe to drop. You don't want them to think you were just buttering them up so you could pounce on them with criticism or complaints.

That's exactly what happened for my client Tiana. Despite my instructions, she couldn't help herself. After complimenting her partner Kelly on her curvaceous body, Tiana blurted out, "I just wish you would let me see you naked more often. I feel like you're always hiding from me because you don't want me to initiate." Kelly accused Tiana of being manipulative with her compliments and shut Tiana down for weeks.

Instead, what you're going to do is give your partner another compliment! It's best if it's something specific they did recently, but you can also call up older memories. Here are some examples:

> "Since we talked about sexual memories last week, I keep thinking about all these great experiences we've shared together. We sure were lucky to have so much chemistry right off the bat."
>
> "I loved that you took a few extra seconds to give me a goodbye kiss yesterday."
>
> "I appreciated that you initiated sex the other day. It made me feel good to know you wanted me."
>
> "I just love looking at your body!"

This step should *not* be used to initiate intimacy. You're still getting your partner used to the idea of talking about sex more openly, and you don't want to make them feel like the only times you talk about sex have to lead to taking your clothes off.

Repeat this step as many times as necessary, until your sex life together starts to feel like a much more comfortable topic. Even then, don't be afraid to keep the compliments flowing. There's no such thing as showing too much appreciation.

The Other Half with Xander: The Fresh Start Conversation

For many people, the steps Vanessa just outlined might feel like too tall an order. Unfortunately, since most people are so embarrassed about sex, they work up the courage to talk about it only when they've allowed issues and resentments to boil over, and things like "You never want me" or "I hate the way you kiss" come tumbling out. As a result, their first (and possibly only) experience talking about sex ends up focused on the *problems* with their sex life rather than the opportunities. And this is a huge mistake, because focusing on the problems tends to lead to fights and hurt feelings, which only further discourage you from talking about sex again in the future. After all, why would you want to talk about something if all you ever do is fight about it?

If sex has been a contentious topic in the past, you may want to have what we like to call a "Fresh Start Conversation." This is your opportunity to have a short, to-the-point talk in which you can simply:

- Acknowledge the past and take ownership for your part. For example, "I know talking about sex has been a challenge for me/us" or "I'm sorry I wasn't open to talking about sex in the past." You can even use Sex Talks to your advantage by saying something like, "I know I have some growing to do, so I bought this book to help me learn to be a better communicator."
- Clear the slate. Tell your partner you want to leave the past in the past and start fresh.
- State your new goals. For example, "I want us to get to a point where we feel comfortable talking openly about sex so we can experience deeper intimacy with each other."

Vanessa and I have had multiple Fresh Start Conversations. While I always felt comfortable talking about sex from an academic perspective with Vanessa, it scared the hell out of me to discuss the nuts and bolts of our own sex life, especially if my body didn't "perform" exactly as I wanted it to. After getting into a particularly negative headspace following a string of lost erections, I initiated my own Fresh Start Conversation by saying, "I know I've shut down in the past and felt uncomfortable talking about what's going on when I have performance issues, but I've been realizing I want to feel like we're on the same team."

The Fresh Start Conversation isn't about litigating the past or making a grand apology; the goal is to acknowledge the reality of your situation and redirect yourselves toward a more positive future. You can even do it via text, just to get the ball rolling. It may take your partner some time to come around to the idea that sex is back on the table as a topic of conversation, but you can create some goodwill by taking ownership of your side of the street.

If All Else Fails, Blame Us!

If you're feeling nervous about talking about your personal sex life as a couple, another option is to start talking about sex *unrelated* to your relationship. Here's the trick: follow us on Instagram and get your partner to do the same. Every single day, Xander and I talk about anything from apologies to fantasies to scheduling sex in our Stories. We also answer tons of questions from our community (if you DM us, we might even pick yours!). You can watch our Stories separately or together, and then have a conversation about our topic of the day. It doesn't matter if the topic doesn't have anything to do with you or your relationship; it's just a conversation opener.

Every day we get feedback from couples in our community about how discussing our posts and Stories was the best way for them to get comfortable talking about sex. That's because it often feels easier to discuss a concept in a more general sense, or a problem another couple is having, versus going immediately into your own experience and the potential emotional baggage or history that goes along with it. After getting comfortable doing this for a while, it starts to feel way easier to mix in talk about your own sex life.

The Post-Game

Now that you've had these experiences with talking about your sex life separate from the act itself, let's up the ante and start the conversation when it's freshest on your mind.

Have you ever watched a post-game wrap-up of a sporting event? A bunch of commentators get together and offer their perspectives on what just happened. You can do this after sex, too—just without all the cheesy graphics and replays. There are some major benefits to talking about sex right after having it:

- It's top of mind. You don't have to start the conversation out of nowhere.
- You've just had a specific experience to discuss and use as an example.
- You're feeling connected to each other.

- You're not operating under any of the pressure most couples feel leading up to and during sex.

For your first Post-Game, zone right in on compliments. Tell your partner that they're a good kisser or that their breasts looked fantastic. Call out the standout moments. For example, "You know that thing you did, where you used both hands on me at the same time? I *really* loved that."

For the second Post-Game, try requesting a repeat for next time. For example, "I liked when you grabbed me and tossed me on the bed. Can you do that again in the future?" This is a great way to ease into making requests of your partner. (I'll go into more detail on requests in another of the Sex Talks, so this is just a teaser.) It feels light and fun, since you're grounding your requests in positive feedback and compliments, but you're still making a specific ask.

Once you're feeling more confident, you can use the Post-Game to ask for something new. The key here is to continue anchoring it with a compliment. For example, "I really liked you telling me how hot I am. What do you think about trying out even more dirty talk next time?"

The only thing to keep out of your Post-Game is criticism. We don't want the sexual equivalent of "Branson really blew that clutch play in the final seconds!" It's just too sensitive a time to bring up anything remotely critical. Instead, focus on what you did like and what you want to try going forward.

The Acknowledgment Transformation

Want to know the coolest thing about the Acknowledgment Sex Talk? It eventually morphs into flirting! This isn't a one-and-done conversation; the benefits extend for much longer.

So many couples ask me how they can recapture the magic of their early days together, and they get particularly nostalgic about all the flirting and banter they used to have. Well, you can't flirt with each other if you can't even acknowledge the act you're hoping that saucy wordplay will lead to! "Hey, Babe, wanna . . . go downstairs and watch *The Office* again?" isn't setting off any fireworks, right?

Because Xander and I are now so open and acknowledging of our sex life, we get to work fun and flirty teasing into our daily life. We can find a way to turn just about anything into a sexual innuendo. It doesn't even have to make sense; just this morning after a random mention of the game Yahtzee, I seductively said to Xander, "I'll roll *your* dice later." It certainly wasn't the sexiest thing I've ever said to him, but it made us both laugh, and it created a tiny moment of intimacy. And it got both of us thinking about being intimate with each other later. (Don't worry, no actual dice were harmed.)

Here are some other ways to turn Acknowledgment into flirting:

- Continue giving each other compliments.
- Reference positive experiences, like "I had so much fun with you last night" or "I can't get what you did out of my head."
- Make suggestive comments or jokes.
- Talk positively about your partner in front of other people.
- Leave little notes for each other. Just something simple—one or two sentences.
- Or send sweet messages as texts.
- Cat-call or wolf-whistle them.

Navigating Common Pitfalls

All the techniques in *Sex Talks* have been tested with my clients and our community, so I'm well aware of some of the unique challenges that can come up. In this section (which you'll find at the end of each of the five Sex Talks), I'll share the stories I've heard of things that went wrong, and how you can protect yourself and your relationship from falling into the same traps.

"We're in the midst of a massive dry spell. It feels extra awkward to try to talk about sex, given that we haven't had it in six months."
The first thing I tell anyone who mentions the phrase "dry spell" is that it's perfectly normal to go through them. When we conducted a casual poll on Instagram, a whopping 93 percent of our followers said that they've had a dry spell in their relationship. Whether they're caused by childbirth, illness, injury, life circumstances, an interpersonal issue, or anything else, please never feel ashamed about being in one.

There isn't an "awkwardness-free" way to get back in the saddle after a dry spell. It's just like when you work out at a gym for the first time in months, or you lead your first meeting after maternity leave: it's bound to feel foreign. But talking about it first, and acknowledging the awkwardness, can help the two of you feel like you're on the same team.

In terms of communication, you've got to rip the bandage off. The longer you go without talking about sex, the harder and harder it will feel to start a conversation.

Tell your partner, "I know our sex life isn't where either one of us wants it to be. I don't know about you, but for me, it feels awkward to talk about it. But I want to have the conversation because I love you, and I care about our intimacy. I'm not saying we need to jump right back into the sack, but could we talk about how to start slowly rebuilding our connection?"

"Sex has never been great in our relationship, even at the beginning. How do I get the Acknowledgment conversation started if I don't have any positive memories to share?"
I'm a firm believer that chemistry can be created, and I've worked with a lot of couples who never had a "honeymoon stage." It's okay if you haven't had any jaw-dropping, earth-shattering experiences with each other. Instead, look for small things to call out, like the way your partner strokes your back

or how good you feel when you're around them. If even that is a challenge, lean on the Blame Us and Post-Game techniques. We'll get you two creating better memories in the fourth Sex Talk.

"I tried casually opening the conversation with my partner a few times, and he got suspicious and asked, 'Why do you keep bringing this up?' I lost my nerve and said 'No reason.'"

Your partner is probably going to notice that you're talking about sex, especially if it's not a regular topic of conversation. That's okay! The goal here is not to secretly get them to talk about sex without their realizing what they're doing. If your partner calls you out in this way, say something like, "I'm realizing that we don't usually talk about sex, even though it's a normal and healthy part of our relationship. I don't have anything specific I want to talk about, but I would like to feel comfortable with it as a topic of conversation."

"My wife doesn't want to talk about our sex life at all. When I've tried in the past, she's said, 'We shouldn't have to talk about our sex life; it should just be natural.'"

That's shame and perfectionism talking. Most of us feel so embarrassed and awkward about sex that we don't want to acknowledge its existence. And the pressure we feel to have perfect, effortless sex makes us feel like something's wrong with us if we have to talk about it. I know it can be frustrating to get this kind of response from your partner, but try to tap into your compassion for them. Imagine how much pressure they're feeling, and how badly they're suffering.

Catch your partner in a quiet moment and say this: "I've heard you say that we shouldn't have to talk about our sex life. I want you to know that I see talking about sex as a way of building intimacy. It makes me feel closer to you to talk about it. It's not about complaining or solving problems; it's just about being able to acknowledge this really special act that we get to share with each other. We talk about every other aspect of our relationship, and I want us to talk about this, too."

Now that you've finally named the elephant in the room and built a solid, positive foundation of sexual communication, let's move on to the next big Sex Talk!

CHAPTER 6

THE SECOND CONVERSATION:
Connection

aka, "What Do We Need to Feel Close to Each Other?"

IT WAS ONE of those nights when we were both trying to pretend we were asleep, but we knew full well that the other person was wide awake. We were both on our sides, facing opposite directions. It was completely silent in the room, but the air was stuffed with all the things left unsaid.

Why doesn't Xander want to have sex with me? I thought, fuming.

Xander and I were in the middle of a particularly busy season of life. Nothing too intense or unusual, just a classic time when we both had packed schedules. We were working far later than we typically did, and we had plans almost every night. The only thing happening in our bed was sleeping—and fuming. At one point, I honestly couldn't remember the last time we had sex. The longer we went without it, the less connected I felt to Xander. The idea of cuddling or kissing on the couch but not having sex afterward felt like too much of a tease, so I pulled away from him more and more. It got to the point where I could feel myself aching for his touch as we crossed paths in the kitchen, but I held my arms behind my back so I wouldn't reach out.

As the disconnection grew, so did my fear and frustration. *Just fuck me already!* I found myself thinking on a daily basis. But I didn't want to be the one to initiate. I wanted to feel *wanted*. I wanted him to *prove* to me that this was just a weird, fluky time in our relationship, and it didn't mean anything scary, like that the spark was fading. I wasn't just horny; I was legitimately scared, frustrated, and angry. And it hadn't dawned on me that having sex with someone who was furious with you might not seem particularly tempting to Xander—or anyone else, for that matter.

———

At the beginning of a relationship, couples often feel pulled to each other like magnets. Closeness feels so easy and natural. It's classic fairy-tale stuff; you'll hear new couples exclaim things like "We're practically the same person!" and "It's like we were made for each other."

But as time goes on, intimacy starts to feel increasingly complex, and this shift is accompanied by a tremendous sense of grief and loss. Why is it so hard to stay connected to the person you love?

In Part One, I talked about becoming a stranger to yourself, and losing your understanding of what you need and desire. Here's how to know whether you and your partner should start your Sex Talks adventure with the Connection conversation: Have you become strangers to *each other*?

Disconnection can take so many different forms: little to no quality time, a dead bedroom, silence, frequent arguments, or a sense of loneliness. But the central theme running through all these dynamics is that feeling of having lost contact with your love.

We tend to think of a relationship as two people merging into one entity. The therapist in me wants to warn you that this isn't a healthy form of intimacy, but the thirteen-year-old girl inside of me remembers singing along to "2 Become 1" by the Spice Girls, and thinking it was the most romantic concept ever. You'll know you need to have the Connection conversation in your relationship if you feel like you have definitively morphed back into two people who feel light-years away from each other.

"I thought being in a relationship would mean I'd never have to be alone again, but now I feel even lonelier in my marriage than I did on my own." My friend Emmy is going through an especially disconnected period with her husband of ten years, Theo. Theo is a college friend of mine, so I knew him before he met Emmy. I remember his giddy, almost childlike excitement when they started dating. Emmy and I became fast friends, and as our individual connection deepened, she started confiding in me more.

"Last night we had this big date night that we had to work so hard to set up. Theo's been working like a maniac, we don't have a reliable sitter ... there are a million other things I won't bore you with. We planned this a month in advance, and it felt like all the stars had to be in alignment, even down to the moment we walked out of the house. And then we get to the restaurant, order our food ... and I literally can't think of a single interesting thing to say to him." Emmy starts to sob. "When we were dating, the conversation was nonstop. It felt like it would be impossible to run out of things to talk about. I remember being on date nights back then, looking around at the sad couples not speaking to each other, and feeling so horrified for them. Now we've *become* one of those couples."

For Emmy and Theo, the predictable things have gotten in the way of their emotional and physical intimacy: kids (including one with serious health issues), demanding jobs, financial stress, and a complete and utter lack of free time. But it goes deeper than that. Even when they battle the logistical challenges and carve out time for each other—like their ill-fated date night—they're hit in the face with the intensity of their disconnection.

"You know how people throw out the phrases like 'roommates rather than partners' and 'ships passing in the night'?" Emmy asks me. "That can't come close to describing how I feel. On good days I look at him and think, *Forget about love. Do I even* like *him anymore?* On bad days I wonder, *Who is this stranger in my home, playing with my children, raiding my refrigerator, using my nice hand lotion?*"

The problem, of course, is that none of us has any freaking clue how to start talking about these incredibly complex dynamics with each other. For Xander and me, our connection had felt so easy and effortless until it didn't. We didn't *have* to talk about intimacy, and that had felt like a good sign! But once we got into a tough place with each other, we didn't have any connection rituals or a communication foundation to fall back on.

Years later, it would shock me to find out that Xander had been just as unhappy as I was during this period of our relationship, only for a completely different reason. And that became the key to us rebuilding our connection and finding our way back to each other.

The Physical-Emotional Conundrum

There are two types of people in the world: people who need to feel emotionally connected in order to have sex, and people who need to have sex in order to feel connected. In a cruel twist of fate, most relationships consist of one of each type. The thing that we need is the reverse of what our partner needs, so a lot of couples feel impossibly stuck.

This is exactly what's happening for Emmy and Theo. Over matcha teas at a busy coffee shop, she hisses under her breath at me: "This motherfucker actually tried to initiate sex last night! I'm still reeling from the date night from hell a few days ago, and he honestly thinks he can just crawl into bed and expect me to open my legs for him? I actually said to him, 'Are you joking?'" She pauses to take an angry gulp. "He looks at me with these sad, puppy-dog eyes, like he can't possibly understand why I wouldn't be into it. So I tell him, 'I can't believe I have to spell this out to you, but I don't want to have sex with you unless I feel *connected* to you!'"

"What was his response?" I ask her, even though I'm pretty sure I already know.

"He says, 'But the way I feel connected to you is by having sex!'"

After going back and forth a few times, Emmy pushing for emotional connection and Theo asking for physical, the conversation stalled out, leaving both of them feeling hopeless.

The Physical-Emotional Conundrum is an incredibly important dynamic for us to understand about ourselves, our partners, and our relationships, so let's unpack what's really going on.

I've mentioned the spark a few times already, and it's a phrase we've all heard over and over, right? The reality is that it's not so much a spark as two twin flames: emotional intimacy and physical intimacy. One can't survive without the other in a long-term relationship.

In that way, Conversations 2 and 3 are sister chapters; this one is about emotional intimacy, and the next is about physical. If left untended, connection and desire both tend to sputter out around the same time in a relationship. It's a chicken-or-egg type of situation, but my hunch is that the connection is the first to go, which is why I'm starting with it here. (There's a second reason why my recommendation is to prioritize emotional intimacy, and I'll share it in a minute.)

In relationships between cis women and men, it's often—but not always—the woman who needs to feel connected first. We did a casual poll of our Instagram audience, and we discovered that 86 percent of women want emotional connection before physical connection, whereas 77 percent of men want the physical connection first. We also asked our audience if this dynamic causes significant tension in their relationship, and 75 percent responded yes.

It wasn't until years later that Xander and I finally understood what had really been going on for us in that "just fuck me already" period of our relationship. In the process of telling Xander about one of the couples I was working with (Ava and Liam—I'll tell you more about them in a bit), I put words to the Physical-Emotional Conundrum for the first time. "It's like she wants to feel emotionally connected first, but he wants to feel physically connected first," I said. "And neither of them is recognizing that, at the end of the day, they're both talking about connection."

"That's exactly what it's like for me!" Xander shouted. "Except I'm like the woman!"

The light bulbs went on. Xander wants connection before sex, but I need sex to feel connected. During our challenging season, Xander had felt so emotionally disconnected from me that he couldn't fathom the idea of being physically intimate. And the lack of physical intimacy created even more emotional distance for me—to the point where I couldn't imagine any other way of reconnecting. But we didn't have the language to explain to each other what we were looking for! At the time, I was stuck in my head thinking, *Why don't you want to have sex with me?* I was more focused on what was going on for Xander than on understanding my own needs and communicating those needs to him. And Xander had been so fixated on my seeming lack of interest in our romantic relationship that he had lost sight of his own emotional needs. We had each become strangers to ourselves, which had led to our becoming strangers to each other. But putting words to the Physical-Emotional Conundrum created a path for finding our way back to each other.

What Is Emotional Intimacy, Anyway?

Whenever we talk about emotional intimacy on Instagram, we get messages like "My husband has the emotional maturity of a can of beans. How can I describe intimacy to him?" Everyone has a different definition, and those definitions can differ based on cultural contexts, but in general, emotional intimacy is a feeling of closeness. You care for each other, and you're willing to use your words and actions to help your partner feel understood, respected, and seen. There's a basic trust that your partner can be a safe container for your feelings and challenges. You feel like you can let down your guard, be vulnerable, and show your true self.

Is Sex Ever Really *Just* About Sex?

Emotional-connection-first types, we need to talk. It's easy for you to write off sex as little more than a physical act, and for your partner's physical needs to feel like an annoyance or a burden. When your partner wants to be intimate with you, it may feel like they're just horny and need a release, and you're merely the vessel. This can be especially true if you're a cis woman in a relationship with a cis man, since there are so many stereotypes of men wanting sex regardless of the circumstances.

But that's not what's really going on for your partner! Even if they seem sex-crazed, they still want to feel emotionally connected to you.

The reason why men are often the ones who want physical intimacy first has a lot to do with socialization. To put it simply, women are given societal permission to be emotional creatures, whereas men are taught that they're not supposed to have feelings. Many of my male clients, even the ones who are more evolved than this caveman-era socialization, have shared with me that the only way they've felt comfortable seeking connection is through sex. Most men simply don't have the capacity to say, "I want to feel close to you right now." I know it might be hard to believe, especially when your partner is buck naked and swinging his penis around like a helicopter, but he's looking for emotional intimacy as much as a physical experience.

The first time I realized this was when I worked with Liam and Ava, a married couple in their late thirties. They owned a business together and had little time in their schedules for connection of any kind. After running into some challenges with their sex life—Liam always wanting more, and Ava feeling exhausted by his needs—Ava had begrudgingly agreed to a compromise: sex twice a week, on Wednesdays and Saturdays. She enjoyed sex on occasion, and sometimes even accepted Liam's initiations on non-scheduled days of the week, but she described sex as mostly "Letting Liam have his way."

He was getting consistent sex, but still, Liam wasn't happy. He was the one who had reached out to set up the session.

"I don't get it," Ava sighed. "It's just not realistic with our schedules for us to have sex more often. But he always said sex twice a week was a healthy frequency, and I've never deprived him of that."

I was a young therapist at the time, and I'll admit that I initially felt as confused as Ava. Ava seemed like a kind and generous partner, and Liam was getting sex far more often than most of my clients. Was he just being greedy? Insatiable? Would anything ever feel "good enough" for him?

"It's not that," Liam said. It was clear that he was struggling with how to phrase what he wanted to say. "I can . . . well, I can tell when you're not into it. And I don't want to have sex with you if that's the case. I don't want 'duty sex' or 'pity sex.'"

"Oh, great, so now I have to be *into it*, too?" Ava asked. "Every time I give you what you want, you set the bar even higher. I feel like I can never keep up. I'll never be able to satisfy you." She started to cry.

"I just want to feel like you're actually *in it* with me!"

It was the word "feel," and the quaver in his voice, that tipped me off.

"Let me tell you what I think is going on here. You guys are both using the word 'sex,' but you're each talking about very different things. Ava, you're talking about sex as a purely physical act, and you're confused almost on a mathematical level. Liam wants sex twice a week, he's getting it twice a week, what's the problem? But Liam, let me guess: If all you wanted was a purely physical release, you have two perfectly good hands for that, right?"

Liam laughed. "I'm not sure I would put it exactly like that, but, yes, you're right."

"What you're actually talking about is wanting to experience connection and closeness with Ava. You want to feel her there in that moment with you. You want it to feel intimate and personal. Like it's Liam and Ava."

"Yes," he said. "Yes, that's exactly it!"

If you're an emotional-intimacy-first type like Ava, and especially if your partner seems to want sex more often than you do, you've probably been way more fixated on the *quantity* than on the *quality* of sex. But I want you to see the common thread that you and your partner are both seeking: those truly vulnerable, intimate moments when time stands still and it's just the two of you. Whether you're having that experience through sex or through some other sort of activity, it's that *connection* you're both truly craving.

So, the next time your partner grumbles, "Yo, wanna do it?" while they scratch the back of their neck, you take a deep breath and picture your partner standing in front of you, their hand on their heart, saying to you, "I love you, and I want to be close to you right now." Does that change how you feel about their desires? (And don't worry; I'll help them learn better initiation techniques in the next chapter!)

Let's Do This

Ask your partner:
  "Do you like to feel emotionally connected first, before having sex? Or does sex feel like your primary way to create emotional connection?"

If your partner wants connection first, ask them:
  "What specific things help you feel connected to me?"
  (We'll get back to this question in a second.)
  "What does sex feel like for you when we have that baseline of emotional connection?"

If your partner wants sex first, ask them:
  "Can you describe to me how sex creates that feeling of emotional connection for you?"
  "How do you feel after sex, as opposed to before?"

Even if we can take this softened approach and recognize the common thread in what we're both looking for, what do we do, logistically, in those moments when one partner wants emotional intimacy and the other wants physical intimacy? Who gets to go first? Someone has to "win," right?

For years after working with Liam and Ava, I tried to encourage couples to focus on their shared desire for connection and to try to meet both partners' needs simultaneously. I advocated for deeper awareness of what each partner was looking for, in the hope that more understanding would lead to less tension.

But I have to be honest and confess that the approach had only limited success, even in my own relationship. I mean, it's kind of a cop-out to say "Just do both!" After many years of reflection, I'm finally ready to take a more definitive stance on the Physical-Emotional Conundrum and say something controversial that not everyone is going to agree with.

Emotional Connection Should Come First

Sex-first types, I hear you. I know it absolutely sucks to hear this. Remember, I'm one of you! (Also, I *really* like winning.) I hated the words the first time I uttered them.

But here's the reality: it often doesn't feel safe or healthy to be physically intimate with someone when you're feeling disconnected from them. When you're dating or having casual sex, emotional connection may not matter as much. But when you have a long-standing relationship with someone, disconnected sex feels pretty icky. If you're a survivor of sexual abuse, this kind of sex can even be triggering or re-traumatizing.

In some of my earlier sessions with Ava and Liam, Ava told me about the worst instances of connection-less sex. "I'd be staring at the ceiling, wishing for him to hurry up and get it over with. It was like he was masturbating into me." Liam didn't like it, either; remember his calling it "pity sex"?

I've even experienced this myself, plenty of times! During challenging seasons of our relationship, I've pushed for Xander and me to have sex in an attempt to rebuild our connection, and Xander went along with it. But it left both of us feeling gross and used. The sex wasn't even remotely fun or pleasurable; we each experienced far more performance issues than we do normally, and it left us feeling even less connected than before. Disconnected sex actually creates even more disconnection.

I've been talking a lot about couples becoming strangers to themselves and each other. When you have sex without emotional connection, it can feel like having sex with a *literal* stranger. For all these reasons, it's more useful to lead with emotional intimacy.

Let me be clear: physical intimacy is equally as important and valid as emotional intimacy. But when you're in a tough place, start with rebuilding the emotional connection first. Which leads us straight into . . .

What Are Your Logs?

We all want to feel close to our partner, right? But let me ask you this: Do you know the *specific* things that help your partner feel connected to you, and the specific things that help *you* feel connected to your partner? What makes the two of you feel like true teammates, as if you're fully in it together? I like to call these your "logs." When the fire burns out in a long-term relationship, it's because we've stopped throwing logs onto the flames. Part of writing your User Manual should be identifying the logs that keep your fire ablaze.

I'm presenting these things as simple questions, but the reality is that connection can often feel surprisingly thorny. At the beginning of my relationship with Xander, it felt like *everything* we did brought us closer together. Watching reruns of *Battlestar Galactica* could feel like a bonding experience, even though I despise sci-fi.

But somewhere along the way the things I needed to feel connected to Xander changed. I didn't notice it until I felt *disconnected*, which made it extra tricky. We needed to come back together as a couple, but we had no clue how to get there.

Even to this day, connection with Xander can feel surprisingly complicated. I can occasionally catch myself feeling confusion, frustration, and even fear, because none of Xander's attempts at connection feel "right." I can tell he's trying to help me feel loved, and I know that I want that, too, but the way he's trying to get there feels so *off*. It leaves me feeling like a cursed version of Goldilocks: "No, that's too hard. No, that's too soft." Except that I never find the "just right."

Even worse, Xander can do the exact same thing that made me feel loved and special the day before, but it doesn't feel bonding to me today. Or he can make a request for something *he* wants to feel connected, and I'll recoil. Sometimes it's because I want a different path to connection, like going on a walk versus watching a movie together. Sometimes what he wants feels like the exact *opposite* thing from what I'm wanting in that moment. Case in point: just twenty minutes ago he asked me for a hug, but I brushed him off with "in a bit" because I was too lost in writing this chapter!

In rare but especially vulnerable moments, these connection challenges evoke an existential type of dread and loneliness within me. How can I feel so alone, even with the person I love the most in this world, and even with him trying *so hard* to connect with me?

Despite all the nuance and gray areas, it's still worthwhile for you and your partner to explore the specifics of what helps you feel close to each other. Yes, "intimacy" might occasionally feel like an enigma that can never be fully solved. But you can—and should—still try. Otherwise, you're just going to feel like you're living life treading water with each other.

So, let's get specific about what makes each of you feel connected. We tend to assume that other people like to give and receive love in the same way that we do. (But as Gary Chapman pointed out in the *Five Love Languages*, this couldn't be further from the truth.)[1] Have you ever had an experience in which you did or said something for your partner that you thought was a big deal, but that your partner hardly acknowledged? Was there ever a time when you did something that seemed minor to you, but your partner's response was over-the-top appreciative? You think that something in particular will mean a lot to your partner because it would mean a lot to you, but that may not be the way they prefer to be shown love. It doesn't mean your partner doesn't appreciate the gesture; it just means that it's not going to be a home run for them.

Xander can make my entire day with four words ("You're killing it, Babe"), but he's bought me some expensive presents that have gone untouched (the funniest was an enormous and uncomfortable pair of white-noise headphones for sleeping).

If you and your partner each know how you each like to give and receive love, you'll have a much better understanding of how to show each other your affection. You know how to push each other's buttons in a negative way, right? How about learning how to push each other's buttons in a positive way, too?

Let's Do This

Ask your partner these questions about their User Manual:

"What are three to five specific things that help you feel connected to me?" (Note that this is a variation of the question from earlier, just getting a bit more specific.)
"What are your three to five favorite ways to receive love?"
"What are your three to five favorite ways to show me your love?"
"If I want to 'push your buttons' in a positive way, what's the best way for me to do it?"

This initial conversation will be a great starting point, and it's also a topic that should be woven into your life. It's your responsibility to keep getting to know what you need when it comes to connection, and to share your discoveries with your partner. This won't always be simple. Your wants are going to be in flux throughout the years, and sometimes you're going to get frustrated by how hard it feels to identify what you need. Life is going to take over, and you're going to feel like you don't have a single second to spare to focus on connection. There will be times when you and your partner will make your best efforts, but you still will wind up stuck in the stranger zone, grappling with that existential fear. You've got to keep fighting your way back to each other, though.

Here's a way to keep it super practical: start every day by asking each other "What do you need to feel connected to me today?" or "How can I support us in feeling close to each other today?" Create a ritual around connection. (I'll also share more tips for ongoing connection in Part Three.)

And make sure to give each other praise and feedback when you get it right, by saying things like "I appreciate your spending this time with me" and "I feel so close to you right now."

For Xander, learning about the Physical-Emotional Conundrum has helped him feel comfortable saying, "I want to feel close to you right now," and just uttering that one sentence makes a surprisingly big difference for him. Even if I'm feeling exhausted or shut down in that moment, it's a gentle reminder to me that I want to be close to him, too. As we do the final edit of this chapter, he reflects on how far he has come in terms of understanding and asking for emotional connection. "There were so many times in the past that I thought I had a low sex drive. Turns out, I'm a horny bastard when I feel emotionally connected to you."

The Bristle Reaction

Let's switch tracks now and talk about physical intimacy. So far, I've been using "physical intimacy" and "sex" interchangeably, but if sex is the only form of physical connection in your relationship, you're going to run into trouble fast. Let me introduce you to the dreaded Bristle Reaction. This is the term I coined for when you feel your entire body recoil when your partner tries to touch you. They could be coming in for a hug, giving you a caress on the back, or trying to kiss you, and you feel yourself tense up. Our familiar stranger archetype surfaces yet again; it's the same sort of reaction you might have if an *actual stranger* tried to touch you.

How the heck does this happen? How can you have such a strong and negative response to the simplest touch from the person you love the most in this world?

Let me tell you the story of Genevieve and Navarro. They're a cisgender heterosexual couple in their early forties with two kids. When they first started dating, they couldn't keep their hands off each other. But like so many couples, they're now in a touch-starved relationship. There's so little physical contact between the two of them that a casual observer might mistake them for good friends.

Navarro has the higher sex drive, so he's typically the partner who initiates most often. Like most people, he feels embarrassed initiating, so he does it in roundabout ways, like trying to extend a hug a bit longer, or trying to slip a little tongue into a kiss. (We'll talk more about initiation in the next chapter.) Navarro just hints at what he wants because, as he admits to me, "If I don't fully put myself out there, it won't hurt as much if Genevieve turns me down."

But Navarro isn't as sneaky as he thinks he is, and Genevieve knows what's up. Over time, Genevieve has become hypervigilant to any sort of touch that feels like it's leading to sex. She doesn't want physical contact to progress too far, because she worries about hurting Navarro's feelings. Just like Navarro secretly thinks it won't hurt as much if he doesn't fully initiate,

Genevieve thinks it won't hurt as much if she turns Navarro down right at the beginning. If she's not interested in sex at the exact moment he tries to slip her a little tongue, she pulls away.

By the time they start seeing me, Genevieve has spiraled down into full-on Bristle Reaction mode. Even when Navarro tries to touch her in small, loving, nonsexual ways, she recoils. Navarro can feel Genevieve pulling away, and it hurts him. He reaches out for her less and less, to the point where the only time Navarro touches Genevieve is to initiate sex.

Which, as you can guess, only further perpetuates Genevieve's hyper-vigilance to Navarro's touch. It reinforces her belief that touch always has a motive and never exists just for simple enjoyment and connection.

It's not that Genevieve wants zero contact. She feels the desire for physical touch, but she doesn't feel comfortable initiating it. She tells me, "Every single time I touch Navarro, he thinks I want to have sex, and will try to turn the contact sexual. Like grabbing my hand and moving it to his crotch. Sometimes I want to just sit close, cuddle, or hold hands without it leading into sex." She sacrifices her own desire for physical contact because she's so afraid it won't be received by Navarro.

And it gets even worse! On the rare occasion that Genevieve agrees to have sex, Navarro tries to get down to business as quickly as possible. He confesses that his reaction in those moments is "Whoa, Genevieve said yes! Better get to it before she changes her mind!" So, Navarro skips over any sort of touch or foreplay and goes straight to intercourse. Which, as you'll learn in a later chapter, is a *huge* problem for cis women.

Do you see the tangled web Genevieve and Navarro have woven?

Now that I've shared Genevieve and Navarro's story, I'm sure you can see how the Bristle Reaction makes perfect sense. But if you've never broken it down in this way before, you've probably thought you're a terrible person if you're a bristler. And it has likely created a huge blockage to communication in your relationship. After all, how can you possibly tell your partner how savage your internal response is to their loving touch? Anytime I post a video about the Bristle Reaction for our audience, we receive hundreds of tearful messages—particularly from women who hadn't realized it was a thing. Genevieve herself told me, "I've felt deep guilt and general torment about this for a very long time. Learning that it's normal and that I'm not alone has been life changing."

I see the Bristle Reaction most often in male-female relationships, but the recoil does not discriminate. My clients Franklin and Willie are a gay couple, and Franklin is a bristler. He shared with me: "I thought this was just me being suspicious AF toward my husband. He totally sneaks in the tongue or the touches, and I bristle up. I don't want it to be like this anymore."

So, how do we fix this complicated dynamic? The best place to start is by incorporating *more* touch into your relationship! You have to break the belief that any sort of touch leads to sex. This will allow both of you to relax and enjoy nonsexual physical connection again.

Nonsexual touch is also an incredible way to break down the physical versus emotional connection dichotomy, since it falls into both realms. Even though I've said that the emotional connection should come first, that doesn't mean you should have zero physical contact until you're feeling deeply in tune with each other. Nonsexual touch increases connection for both partners and helps the physical-first partner feel seen and respected.

Exercise: Touch Time

One of the best things you can do for your relationship is to create structured "touch time," when you're *only* engaging in nonsexual touch. Let's be super clear: the point of this time is *not* to get turned on and then want to have sex. It's to enjoy touch *just* for the sake of touch! Sometimes I even tell couples, "I don't care if you both wind up getting turned on and wanting to have sex. *Do not* have sex right after your touch time!"

Every day, set aside at least five minutes for your nonsexual touch time. (You can even turn it into a sweet ritual by always doing it at the same time, or setting up your space in a special way.) This is your opportunity to unwind, to connect with each other, and to learn to enjoy the simple pleasures of touch.

For example, Xander and I spend five minutes cuddling in bed at the end of every night. It has become a habit, so now we don't even need to think about it. You can even come up with a funny name for it; Xander and I use "skin-to-skin," or "STS."

Exercise: The Thirty and Six

There are two forms of physical touch that have been scientifically proven to lead to deeper connection: the thirty-second hug and the six-second kiss. Oxytocin—otherwise known as the "cuddle hormone" or the "love hormone"—makes us feel relaxed, trusting, and connected to our loved ones. It gets released after twenty to thirty seconds of touch and about six seconds of kissing. If you want a simple way to add more connection to your relationship, make the space for one thirty-second hug and one six-second kiss every day.

What to Do When You Feel Completely Touched Out

Even though touch is wonderful and can be a great way to create more intimacy and connection, we all have a limit for how much we can take. There's even a term for it: being "touched out." You don't want to be touched, regardless of the intent behind the contact. It's a cousin of the Bristle Reaction.

Primary caretakers can get touched out after being in physical contact with their kids all day long. You've been touched, poked, prodded, latched onto, and grabbed at for hours, and the thought of having any more physical contact makes your skin crawl. If you have a baby, they may literally rely on your body for nourishment and comfort, and you may be in skin-to-skin contact with them the majority of the day. If you've recently given birth, you may feel disconnected from your body, which can further complicate the sensation of being touched out.

While people most frequently refer to feeling touched out because of kids, you can also experience it from physical contact with your partner, someone you're taking care of, or even clingy pets. (Any fellow pug owners will know exactly what I mean.)

Being touched out is awful in and of itself, but it also makes connection with your partner feel even more complicated. Let's say you've been watching the kids all day, and your partner comes home from work and wants a big hug, or wants you to cuddle on the sofa with them for a few minutes, or wants to have sex. Even if you love your partner—and even if you love physical intimacy with them—you may find yourself recoiling. Vivian from our Instagram community messaged me to say, "I feel like I give to everyone all day long, so at the end of the day when it could be time to be intimate, I just don't have the energy left to give of myself. I feel touched out and tired and not cared for, so I just want to have quiet space and not have to give anymore."

Despite recognizing how intense this experience can be, so many people still ask me, "How do I get turned on after a long day of being touched out?" But here's the thing: you can't be touched out and turned on at the same time. Being touched out means you're past capacity. It's your body's cry for help. Being a parent or caretaker is incredibly demanding, and it's normal to feel emotionally overwhelmed by how much you're needed.

Imagine that you've just had a huge meal and you've hit the "unbuttoned *and* unzipped my pants" level of stuffed. If your partner offers you food, you're probably not going to want it, right? Even if your partner offers you your absolute favorite meal, the idea of taking another bite isn't going to sound very tempting. You get the comparison I'm making, right? But let's be honest—when your partner initiates sex these days, do you often anticipate getting the sexual equivalent of the meal of your life, or of a barely defrosted Lean Cuisine?

The bottom line is that if you're feeling touched out, you need more support. You're probably not going to get to a place where you *never* feel touched out, but you can definitely lessen the frequency and intensity. "Getting more support" can mean a lot of different things, and I know it's something *far* easier said than done. But one of the most effective solutions is to prioritize alone time for yourself every day. You need the opportunity to come home to your body and reconnect with yourself before you can connect with anyone else. A 2018 survey found that, on average, parents have only thirty-two minutes per day to themselves.[2] Whatever it takes, try to get more alone time. Even if all you can manage some days is one extra minute, that's something. If you have a decent chunk of time, try to do an activity involving your body, like taking a nap, going for a walk around the block, or dancing to your favorite song. If you have only sixty seconds to spare, close your eyes and take slow, deep breaths. A little sensory deprivation can work wonders when you're overstimulated.

You and your partner need to be teammates, supporting each other in getting this much-needed alone time. Your self-care should be just as important to your partner as their own. You also need to ask for more household support from your partner. Regardless of how you and your partner split up the duties, they need to support you in managing and avoiding burnout.

A lot of people are hesitant to talk to their partner about feeling touched out because they're worried about hurting their partner's feelings. But your partner already knows something is up. And what do you think is worse for them—feeling you physically recoil from them with no idea why, or feeling you recoil but understanding that it's not personal? It can help to walk them through a day in the life of your body. Describe all the different times and ways it has been grabbed, poked, and needed.

Finally, you need to make sure you're having sex that is *for you*, not just for your partner. Your enjoyment and pleasure have to be equally important. As Clara from our Instagram community put it, "I need touch that is *giving*, not *taking*. I get *taking* touch all day long." We'll get to this in later chapters, but if sex feels one-sided, it's understandable you'd want to withdraw from it.

The Other Half with Xander: Mental Load and Choreplay

If the idea of talking to your partner about burnout and getting more of their support feels scary, let me introduce you to a concept that might help you feel a bit more motivated: Mental Load. It's the invisible mental burden of keeping track of household needs. And I'm not just talking about the chores! It's the brain power and capacity needed to plan, organize, and reshuffle everything that needs to be done for the maintenance of a family or home. Mental Load never ends, and often it feels inescapable. Unlike a traditional job, where you can leave your work at the office (or at the very least have the option to snooze notifications on your phone), Mental Load can rear its ugly head at literally any moment of the day. For example, "Uh-oh—that's the end of the cereal! It's on back order with Amazon, so I'm going to need to stop by the store to buy more today. We can probably squeeze in a stop after soccer practice, but I'll have to call Aimee's mom to let her know I'll be dropping her off later than usual. Wait, wasn't Joey complaining about the cereal being off-brand? Should I cave in and buy the name brand? And if I'm going to the grocery store today, that means I could also get . . ." (Should I stop here, or keep going?)

We all carry some amount of Mental Load, but the frustrating reality is that women in particular have been socialized to carry the Mental Load—in addition to the majority of the household duties—in most relationships. And this tends to be the case even when a male-female couple is explicit about not wanting to have stereotypical gender roles in their relationship.

Carrying the bulk of the load can have a huge impact on physical and emotional intimacy. When we first started posting about Mental Load on Instagram, Mychelle commented: "I'm nine months postpartum, and we've been struggling hard. I'm overwhelmed with working full time, managing the house, baby, animals, and everything else. I have so much on my plate. It makes me resentful to watch him lie on the couch until noon on his days off while I'm on the go constantly."

While you won't ever be able to do away with Mental Load completely, it will hold less power over you if you discuss your experience with your partner and talk about ways to share it. Plus, you might even have more sex! A 2016 Cornell University study found that couples who shared housework in a way that felt more even had more frequent and enjoyable sex than couples in which the woman did most of the chores.[3]

Splitting up the housework might even turn one or both of you on. There are a lot of jokes out there about how "porn for straight women" is just a bunch of videos of men vacuuming or doing the dishes. But seeing their partner doing certain chores or taking care of things without being asked can be a surprisingly huge turn-on for a lot of people of all genders. In fact, there's even a name for it: choreplay. Vanessa *loves* a freshly made bed, so I try to make a point of expertly tucking in the top sheet when I know she's looking. I can even turn it into a playful initiation by saying, "Hey, Babe, come check out what I did in the bedroom!"

The Strangers

If you've read this far, it's safe to say that you want real intimacy in your relationship. But are you truly willing to do what it takes to get it?

Connection isn't a tank you fill up once, or a destination you arrive at and never leave. Throughout the course of your relationship, you will lose yourselves and each other countless times. You will look at the person you've become, and the person your partner has become, and not be able to recognize either. Are you willing to keep looking for yourself and each other, over and over again?

My friend Emmy isn't. She asks for a trial separation from Theo as I'm writing this book. "I'm too tired," she tells me. "It's too hard." I don't believe in soulmates, and I don't believe every relationship is worth fighting for. But I do suspect that in Emmy's case, she's walking away because of her own discomfort with vulnerability, not because they're incompatible.

Navigating Common Pitfalls

"It feels weird to have to ask my fiancée for the specific things that make me feel connected. If I have to ask for it, it feels like it doesn't count."

The Fucking Fairy Tale teaches us that our partner should always magically know what we want, so a lot of people feel embarrassed or shy to ask for what they need, even with their own partner. But your partner is not a mind reader. As well as you might know each other, they're never going to know what you want 100 percent of the time. Asking for something doesn't take away the value of it! For example, let's say you tell your partner that getting flowers makes you feel loved. A bouquet doesn't instantly appear in your partner's hands the moment you say that. They still have to take the time and make the effort to get it for you. The value isn't lost simply because you spoke the words "I'd love flowers" out loud.

Plus, your taking the time to identify the specific words and actions that make you feel emotionally connected is a great and necessary act of self-discovery.

"I need physical touch and relaxation before jumping into sex, but my partner isn't a cuddler. I get worried that asking him to be more proactive with cuddling will just end up making it feel inauthentic or like a chore that he doesn't want to do."

Xander and I have this dynamic in our relationship, too; he's a huge cuddler and I'm not. If he didn't ask me to cuddle, I could probably go days without thinking about it. Cuddling just isn't something that comes "naturally" to me. But I hate the word "inauthentic," especially as it pertains to sex. There are tons of inauthentic things we do in our relationships—inside and outside of the bedroom. It doesn't matter if I'm not a natural or authentic cuddler. I know that Xander loves it, and I love doing things that make him feel loved.

Tell your partner, "I know you're not a natural cuddler, and I completely respect that. I'm not asking you to be the exact same person I am. But I would love it if you made the effort to cuddle me so I can feel closer to you. I'll make an effort to remind you regularly, since I know it's probably not something that's going to be top of mind for you."

"I tried talking about emotional intimacy with my partner, and he said, 'We shouldn't have to work this hard at it. You know I love you. Why should I have to do all this stuff?' I didn't know how to respond, so the conversation hit a dead end."

Emotional intimacy isn't a one-and-done thing! It's not like you give your partner one compliment or have one deep conversation, and now you're bonded for life. Intimacy is a series of daily decisions made over and over again.

If your partner feels resistant to talking about emotional intimacy, tell them that the continual effort is what feels meaningful to you. Ask them, "Would you expect us to have sex just once, and feel intimately connected for the rest of our lives? Of course not! Emotional intimacy works the same for me."

"I want to have more nonsexual touch time with my wife, but if we start touching each other, and I don't immediately get hard, she gets upset. She says she feels like I'm not attracted to her."

If you're concerned about sexual arousal, and what it looks like for you, our discussion of nonconcordance on page 43 might be interesting to you. But the bottom line is that nonsexual touch is supposed to be . . . nonsexual. The point is to break the connection between touch and sex, eliminate the Bristle Reaction, and have more physical and emotional intimacy in your relationship! Tell your partner, "The hardness of my penis isn't the defining signal of how attracted I am to you. Plus, I want us to have touch with each other that doesn't feel sexual."

JUST THE TIP(S):

- It's shockingly hard to stay emotionally connected in a long-term relationship.
- The spark isn't really just a spark. It's twin flames: emotional intimacy and physical intimacy.
- Emotional disconnection can take so many different forms: little to no quality time, a dead bedroom, silence, frequent arguments, or a sense of loneliness.
- There are two types of people in the world: those who need to feel connected in order to have sex, and those who need to have sex in order to feel connected. You're probably one type, and your partner is probably the other.
- But sex is rarely ever just about sex (especially for cis men, despite the stereotypes). Sex is still a form of connection.
- Emotional intimacy and physical intimacy are equally important; however, when a couple is struggling with disconnection, emotional intimacy should come first.
- It's our ongoing responsibility to identify our Connection needs and share them with our partner, and vice versa.
- The Bristle Reaction is when you feel your entire body recoil when your partner tries to touch you. Nonsexual touch is the key to resolving it.
- The challenges of Mental Load and being touched out can also impact intimacy.

Once emotional intimacy is starting to feel stronger, it's time for the next big conversation!

CHAPTER 7

THE THIRD CONVERSATION:

Desire

aka, "What Do We Each Need to Get Turned On?"

FLICK

I watch the balled-up booger soar from the tips of Xander's fingers, straight over to my side of the bed, landing just inches from my face.

"*Babe!*" I yell.

He looks up at me, startled, his index finger still deeply penetrating his nostril. (Apparently this man just loves putting his fingers in things . . .)

Have you ever had those moments in a relationship when you look at your beloved partner and think, *How could I possibly ever want to have sex with you again?*

So many beautiful memories spring to mind for me. The time I woke up in the middle of the night to the sounds of Xander sleepwalking to the bathroom and peeing all over himself. The time I watched him eat a bag of chips and lick his fingers clean, after pumping gas and not washing his hands afterward. The countless times he's given me a full play-by-play of his "rough session" on the toilet.

Ah, the joys of long-term relationships! It's no wonder that getting turned on feels like a superhuman task sometimes. (Or maybe it feels this way for your partner.)

I'm being funny because I'm trying to ease us into one of the most challenging conversations for couples to have about their sex lives: the disappearance of desire in a long-term relationship. As I mentioned in Part One, sex drive is one of the top three topics that pop up in our DMs and emails. So many people think they *should* be having more sex, but most of them don't actually *want* to be doing it more often. Many people feel wildly disconnected from their libido, like it's some complex code they just can't crack—and frankly, they are too exhausted to even attempt.

What makes this all the more complicated is that the Fucking Fairy Tale rears its ugly head again. We're led to believe that sex drive is an indicator that we have good chemistry with someone, and that we should leave a relationship if it's not there initially or it starts to sputter later on. We're taught that we're supposed to feel desire naturally and spontaneously, and that we shouldn't need to *do* anything to feel desire. And it often feels that way at the beginning of a relationship, so we never wind up talking about what turns us on.

Even though sex drive is something you experience in your own body (that's why we started with the "Me" in Part One), it often has a lot to do with what's going on between you and your partner (the "We"). That's what makes the conversation so tricky to have. It's hard enough to admit to your partner, "I feel like a husk of my formerly sexy self. I can't remember the last time I felt the desire to feel pleasure in my own skin." It's even harder to tell your partner, "*You're* part of the reason why I don't want to have sex." How do you tell the love of your life that their poor hygiene habits are making it hard for you to want to go in for a kiss? Or that you're so resentful about their not doing their fair share of the chores in your relationship that you're purposefully withholding sex as a punishment?

I can laugh about Xander's snots now that I'm safely out of the flick zone, but the reality is that those freaking boogers have a real impact on my desire for him. Pretty much *everything* he says and does has an effect on my desire for him—even things that don't seem immediately related to sex: the way he carries himself, his tone of voice, how much he gets done in a day. Sometimes even how heavily he's breathing! How do I tell him that without making him feel like he's constantly being observed and judged? How do I acknowledge the impact he has on me without sending myself into a shame spiral about the things I must do that erode his attraction to me? (I later asked Xander, and he said: "When you play my belly like a drum, when you refer to my dick as my 'weenis' or 'penne,' the way you scratch yourself when you have bug bites . . . Should I keep going? This feels like a loaded question.") I can get hyper-fixated on the things Xander does that turn me *off*, but the reality is that Xander's *not* picking his boogers isn't going to make me want to rip off my clothes, either.

There are so many ways that arousal can get tricky. If you've never had a conversation about what turns you on, how do you work up the nerve to share that information with your partner for the first time after years or even decades together? How do you tell your partner that the things that were surefire turn-ons for you at the beginning of your relationship don't really do it for you anymore? What if you're embarrassed by what you need to get turned on? What if it feels like *nothing* seems to turn you on anymore? There's a lot to unpack here.

Every couple should talk openly about what they need to get turned on, but this conversation will be an especially important one if sex has lost any of its appeal for you. You need this Sex Talk if the things your partner does to try to initiate intimacy or turn you on just aren't working, or if your partner is actively turning you *off*, or if it feels like you're playing a game of cat and mouse with each other—one partner always pursuing, the other always running away.

We're going to go on a grand adventure together, tracing a sexual interaction from the moment one partner starts to get the slightest inkling that they'd like to be intimate to navigating whether or not you're actually going to have sex. We'll talk about Initiation Styles and Sex Menus and the Sex Drive Simmer versus Turn-On Time. While we'll refer back to your User Manual from time to time, we'll mostly focus on you and your partner working together. Because, ultimately, desire is a team sport in a long-term relationship.

Sharing Your "Me"

Just to quickly recap, in Part One, we talked about:

- The two sex drive types: Spontaneous and Responsive. Remember that Spontaneous types feel mental desire first, then their physical arousal follows. Responsive types are the exact opposite; the physical arousal comes first, then the mental desire second.
- Reverse and Drive mode. Your Reverse dynamics actively take you out of the mood, and your Drive dynamics put you in the mood.

Let's Do This

Now it's time to loop back around and share what you learned with your partner. I like starting this way with couples because it builds goodwill and trust in your relationship. You're taking responsibility for your side of the street and showing your partner that you're willing to take action.

Here's your framework for what to say to your partner: "Our relationship and our sex life are important to me. I wanted to be proactive, so I did some research. This is what I discovered about my sex drive and what I need to do to keep my engine revving.

Here's what I'm going to do about it, and here's what you can do to support me." Keep the emphasis on yourself for now. (Remember that we're in the Sharing Your "Me" section.)

If you're nervous about this, you don't even have to use the words "sex drive." You can simply say, "These are the things that get in the way of our intimacy." That simple word swap can feel a lot more comfortable.

Serene and Jarron are in their early thirties and have four kids. Jarron works long hours at a demanding job so that Serene can be a stay-at-home mom. Their support system is limited because they moved for Jarron's job, and they have no family nearby and only a few work acquaintances for friends.

Their relationship was never that hot and heavy to begin with, which worries them both. Serene asks me: "Aren't relationships supposed to have a honeymoon stage, and *then* things drop off? Is it bad that we never had that phase?" Still, both of their sex drives have decreased significantly in the last year, to the point where they're averaging once every three to four weeks, if they're lucky.

Serene has a slightly higher drive than Jarron does. She believes men are supposed to think about sex constantly, so it makes her self-conscious that Jarron doesn't seem to want her that often. It doesn't feel like there's any sort of an electrical charge between them during day-to-day life, and when one of them is interested in having sex, they don't know how to get the other excitedly on board. Sex typically gets initiated by one of them saying, "It's been a while...should we?" But when they do have sex, they both enjoy it, which leaves them confused about why it doesn't happen more often.

I do individual sessions with each of them, and we uncover a number of understandable reasons why their sex drives have plummeted. That's almost always the case. I know it can be scary when your sex drive decreases, but it's rare that I don't uncover identifiable reasons for the change. The solution to bringing your sex drive back may not be simple or easy, but for my clients it's a huge relief to know that there are specific causes. You weren't abducted by aliens in the middle of the night, and they didn't suck out your sex drive before transporting you back to your bed.

In a joint session, we go over their "Me" dynamics. For Jarron, it's the greatest hits: work stress, not taking care of his body, and performance anxiety. Serene is on antianxiety medication, which has done wonders for her mental health, but it may be the culprit for her lower libido.

The atmosphere in the room feels lighter than it has in previous sessions. I wouldn't describe either of them as happy, but there's little tension because there's nothing to argue about. They're each just sharing their truth, in an act of joint vulnerability.

That is, until Serene starts talking about her body. "It hasn't been the same since the kids. The stretch marks, the scars, the apron belly. My breasts are halfway to the floor. It's just not a pretty look." She starts to cry. "*I* wouldn't want to have sex with me."

Jarron looks at her with so much tenderness that I start to choke up. Simply, but with conviction, he tells her, "I love your body."

"You're just saying that to be nice," Serene says, wiping her eyes with a tissue. It's obvious they've had this conversation before. I want to keep the focus on their "Me" dynamics, but a question pops into my head that I can't resist asking.

"Jarron, what do you see when you look at Serene's body?"

"I see my *wife*. My best friend. The love of my life. Not the collection of individual body parts and 'flaws' that she just rattled off." He takes a deep breath, gathering steam. "I don't see just her body; I see a story behind every part of it. That body gave me my kids. That body survived anxiety attacks. That body climbed mountains with me. She's perfect just the way she is." Jarron reaches out and grabs Serene's hand.

We're just beginning the work, but this is the beautiful thing about talking about sex openly. Serene and Jarron haven't even made any changes to their sex life yet, but they're being truly vulnerable with each other for the first time in ages, and that's already creating the kind of intimacy they've both been starving for.

Moving On to the "We"

Unlike the "Me" dynamics of sex drive, which are your responsibility, the "We" dynamics are things that the two of you can work on together. Let's talk about how to take a team approach to desire.

When I asked our community on Instagram why they struggle to talk about sex drive with their partners, the most common response I got was: "It's easy to fall into the blame game of whose fault it is that we're not having very much sex." But your sex life is not the responsibility of just one partner. Sex is a team sport, and so is getting in the mood for it! One partner's libido only *feels* like an issue if your sex drives are different. If you're the lower-desire partner, it's likely that you get criticized for not wanting sex "often enough." But you could turn around and tell you partner, "Your sex drive is too high. You need to work on lowering it by yourself." Would that feel very good for either of you? Of course not. (Also, let me take a moment to state that my goal is to show you how to unlock your desire potential, not to perpetuate the myth that everyone needs to have a sky-high libido. There is no such thing as a "right" or "normal" sex drive.)

Don't Men Always Want It More?

Like Serene, most people think that men always want more sex than women in cis male-female relationships. Can you think of a single example from a TV show or movie, or even a book, of a heterosexual relationship in which the woman had a higher sex drive? But we recently asked our Instagram audience who had the higher libido in their cis male-female relationship, and 46 percent of respondents said it was the woman! You need to know that this damaging myth is wrong, and that it's perfectly normal and common to be in a male-female relationship in which the woman is the partner with the higher drive.

The best way for you and your partner to work together as a team is to do what I like to call the Sex Drive Simmer. Later in this chapter, we'll get into the specifics of how to get turned on in the moment, but the Sex Drive Simmer is a way of creating the *potential* for desire to arise in the first place. Most of us think about getting turned on only in the moments before having sex, but how you interact with each other throughout the day deeply affects your level of desire for each other. Here's a way to dramatically reframe your approach to sex: the minute you finish having sex is when you begin foreplay for the next time! Think about trying to boil a pot of water. If you start with ice-cold water, it's going to take forever to heat up. You're going to catch yourself staring at the stove, wondering if it will *ever* get warm, debating if you actually *want* the pasta you were going to cook in it. But if you keep a pot of water on a low simmer all day, you can get up to a boil right away. Sex drive works the same way, especially for Responsive types.

I ask Serene and Jarron: "What do you think the Sex Drive Simmer could look like for the two of you?"

Serene looks at Jarron. "I just love the fact that we're talking about this together, as a couple. I don't feel so alone anymore. I think a lot of it for me is feeling like we're in a good place emotionally."

Jarron squeezes her hand. "This is making me think about the beginning of our relationship. You're right, Vanessa, about the foreplay thing. It felt like everything we did back then was foreplay. More touching, kissing, flirting. I was always leaving her little love notes. Sometimes they were a little more, uh, *explicit* than your standard love note." They exchange a knowing glance and start laughing.

"I forgot about those!" Serene exclaims. "Those letters really turned me on."

I jump in. "Okay, so maybe the romantic love notes fall into Simmer territory, but the saucy ones are straight-up 'As soon as I see this, I'm going to get turned on'?" Serene nods her head.

Jarron continues, "We were religious about date night every week. We winked at each other all the time. Serene would slap my ass. Little things like that. Exactly like what you're saying; a slap on the butt isn't enough to get me horny in the moment, but it keeps that sexual energy alive between us. I don't know why we stopped doing all that."

I can see the gears turning in both their brains.

"We can get that simmer going again!" Serene smiles at Jarron.

Let's Do This

Discuss with your partner how the two of you can keep the Sex Drive Simmer going in your relationship. Once you have this conversation about teamwork and the Sex Drive Simmer under your belt, it's time to turn to one of the trickier conversations: the things that shut down your desire altogether.

Talking to Your Partner About Your Turn-Offs

We asked our Instagram audience, "What's something your partner does that *instantly* turns you off?" and we got these responses:

"Trying to kiss me with coffee breath."

"Mansplaining."

"Getting drunk."

"Initiating by pulling out the lube and tossing it at me."

"Just getting naked. No. I need a little romance first."

"When I bend over to pick something up, he comes up behind me and grinds himself against my ass *every time*."

"Complaining about how long it's been since we last had sex."

"Deep throat and phlegm clearing." (This is such a turn-off for me that just typing it is nauseating.)

Burping and farting. (Okay, this is my personal addition. Nothing turns me off faster. And if it's a smelly one? *Forget about it*.)

"When he eats yogurt it's *so loud*. Like, *how*?! Yogurt is such a quiet food to eat!"

"Referring to having sex as 'doing it.'"

I don't care if you're married to Scarlett Johansson; something your partner says or does is going to be an instant, one-way ticket to turn-off-ville. So, how the heck do you tell your sweetie that they're driving you wild—in the wrong way?

First, I gotta put in another plug for leading with the emotional connection. Remember that this Sex Talk and the last one are sisters. Your baseline level of connection dictates how much these small annoyances chip away at your attraction. When Xander and I are in a great place, I can roll my eyes when he lets the burps fly. Sometimes I can even laugh. But when things feel tense between us, I can smell chips on his breath from a football field away, and it makes me want to scratch my eyeballs out and never let him see me naked ever again. When your connection tank is full, you're a whole hell of a lot more patient.

Otherwise, focus on the things your partner does that *do* turn you on. There's almost always a way to reframe something negative to focus on the positive. (We'll take this same tactic in the next chapter, with the section "Positively Pleasurable Feedback.") For example, "You look so sexy when you put on a fresh, tight white T-shirt" instead of "I can't believe you're wearing that sweat-crusted, baby vomit–flecked tank top for the fourth day in a row." Remember that for many of us, Reverse dynamics are more easily identifiable than Drive ones. If you can easily identify your turn-offs, you can back into your turn-ons.

If there's something specific your partner does that you just can't figure out how to reframe, bring it up at a completely separate time, when the two of you are calm and relaxed. It's important to be gentle. You don't want your partner thinking that you're blaming, criticizing, or insulting them. For example, your partner will probably get defensive if you blurt out something like, "I was exhausted because you didn't help with the kids last night, so why on earth would I want to have sex with you?" Instead, tell your partner something like, "Hey, can I talk to you about something sensitive? I know we've been talking about our sex life lately, and I have good news! I identified a pretty simple and straightforward thing you could do to help me feel more desire: keep the door closed when you're going to the bathroom. You know what they say about keeping a little mystery alive in a relationship...."

The Connection Between Enjoyment and Desire

Let's bring the sex drive conversation home by touching on the *quality* of sex you're having. A lot of people judge themselves for having a low sex drive, but most people fail to make the connection between their *desire* for sex and their *enjoyment* of it. I need you to be brutally honest with yourself about the quality of the sex that you're having. Is it sex that is *worth* craving?

Whenever I ask people to describe what sex is like in their relationship, I hear things like "Sex feels so blah, but I don't know how to make it better" and "Sex is almost always one-sided." If the sex that you're having is boring and predictable, if there's nothing in it for you, if you're not experiencing very much pleasure, then *why on earth* would you crave it? It wouldn't make any sense to! Do you ever get wildly excited to eat a bowl of so-steamed-it's-turning-to-mush broccoli? Are you ever jumping-up-and-down thrilled to read the back of a shampoo bottle? Of course not! Sex isn't any different.

We'll get back to this dynamic in greater detail in Conversation 5 (where I'll refer to it as the White Toast Problem), but the good news is that you can feed two birds with one scone here: by focusing on having higher-quality sex, you can increase your desire *and* your pleasure!

All Systems Go: Turn-On Time

Let's say you and your partner have kept that Sex Drive Simmer going, and now you're wanting to turn it up to boil and actually start having sex. Unfortunately, this is another point where most of us come to a screeching halt. Let me tell you about my clients Jacee and Blue. They're a child-free couple who have been married for eight years. (Jacee is nonbinary and uses the pronouns "they" and "them.") Jacee and Blue average sex once a month, and neither is happy about it. As I get to know more about each of them and their relationship, it doesn't seem to me that there's a problem with either of their sex drives. The issue seems to be about getting sex going in the moment.

Jacee tells me that they have a lot on their plate: they're pursuing a degree in social work, working two different jobs with unusual hours, and volunteering with at-risk LGBTQQI teens. They spend almost all their time helping others, and the thought of coming home and then needing to expertly seduce Blue feels exhausting.

Blue lets out a deep breath and chimes in. "It's not just Jacee struggling here. I know this is really dysfunctional and the definition of cutting your nose off to spite your face, but when we're going through a dry spell, I don't want to be the first to crack. I want Jacee to initiate. But then I get self-conscious that they don't want me, we become more distant from each other, and we both want less sex as a result. It's a vicious cycle."

The Inescapable Pain of Rejection

In the early stages of our work together, we discover that Jacee and Blue are both Responsive types, and they each keep waiting for the other to take the lead and initiate sex. I'm always eager to tell my clients about Responsive sex drive, since it's so misunderstood, and I'm anticipating an enthusiastic response from each of them. I get it from Blue ("Oh, that explains so much!"), but Jacee stays quiet. My therapeutic Spidey sense starts to go off, and I just know that something else is up. I gently push Jacee to share any other reasons why they rarely initiate. They finally confess, "Honestly, I'm *terrified* to initiate sex with Blue. I hate rejection and I'm so afraid she's going to turn me down." Growing up nonbinary in a binary world has been tough for Jacee, and they're particularly sensitive to rejection.

I tread carefully. "None of us enjoys being turned down. And I can appreciate that you've had experiences with rejection that most people can't even fathom. It's important for us to talk about this, because rejection is part of the price of admission for a healthy sex life."

When it comes to sex, someone always has to step up and get it started. As much as you may dream of having those magic fairy-tale moments when you just *look* at each other in the right way and it's on, sex in a long-term relationship almost always requires a more active initiation. One person needs to get the ball rolling.

And initiating *always* feels vulnerable because it means putting yourself in the position to be turned down. Xander could be lying naked on the bed with a raging boner, and I would still occasionally find myself feeling a little awkward asking if he wants to do something with said boner.

If you think about it, there are few things in life in which we run the risk of being turned down so often. Rejection is a deeply uncomfortable feeling, and most of us have taken great pains to avoid it.

Plus, it can feel even more complicated if you don't understand the interplay between sex and connection. In the moment, you might initiate sex because you want to feel close to your partner, but they might think what you're really saying is, "I want to have a physical release and you're a convenient way for me to achieve that."

The bottom line is this: you and your partner are different people, and despite your best efforts, you're not always going to feel open to sex on the same day or in the same way. I'm not saying that being turned down is ever going to feel good. But it's something we all need to learn how to manage.

The Initiation Dance

People deal with their fears of rejection in one of two ways: by rarely initiating sex (like Jacee and Blue), or by trying to turn initiation into a joke using techniques like the dreaded Boob Honk. You know, when one partner comes up behind their boob-having partner, reaches around, and squeezes the breasts like a couple of old-school bicycle horns? Never in my entire career have I met someone who responded to the Boob Honk by saying, "Hell yes, rip off my clothes and let's go have sex right now!" But people keep trying to get intimacy going in these roundabout ways because initiating sex makes us feel so vulnerable. If you initiate half-heartedly, or "as a joke," then it won't hurt as much if your partner says no. After all, you were only playing around! The problem is, of course, that having sex initiated in this way doesn't feel like the exciting invitation that initiation should be. (And remember that it also leads to the Bristle Reaction.)

The Worst Initiation Techniques

Just to make sure we don't leave any stone unturned, here's a list of some of the worst initiation techniques I've heard about from my clients (and have even experienced myself . . . [cough, cough] . . . Xander!).

The Random Humper: You sneak up behind your partner and start thrusting against their butt or leg, like a dog in heat. Typically when your partner is engaged in another activity, like washing the dishes or bending over to pick up toys.

The Look Giver: You try to give your partner a "sexy look," but it usually ends up looking like you just have some lint in your eye.

The Hand Kidnapper: You grab your partner's hand and not so subtly move it onto your crotch.

The Scorekeeper: You keep detailed and specific records of exactly how often you and your partner have sex, and make sure you reference the data when you initiate. ("Come on, it's been two weeks!")

The Sleep Interrupter: You wake your partner up after they've already drifted off to sleep (or even in the middle of the night) to get it on.

The Slapper: You proudly whip out your erection and whack it against your partner's body. (Variant: *The Show-Off:* Proudly brandishing your erection without the slapping. Perhaps a helicopter movement?)

The Dramatic Sigher: You make loud and disgruntled sighs that you expect your partner to interpret as an initiation (or to cue them to initiate).

The Other Half with Xander: Isn't It the Man's Job to Initiate?

When it comes to initiating sex in male-female relationships, there are some outdated gender dynamics that tend to harm us. Cis dudes are taught that "real men" need to be assertive, even aggressive. We're supposed to always want sex, and therefore not show any hesitation or lack of confidence in initiating it. And when we do take the lead, we're celebrated by our male friends for going out and "getting it." Cis women, on the other hand, aren't supposed to want too much sex—and if they do, they tend to get labeled as "slutty."

I've experienced all these dynamics firsthand. In college, despite finding myself more attracted to women who were sexually confident and assertive, I worried about being made fun of for dating someone my male friends might see as "too promiscuous." Regretfully, I chose not to date or kept hookups secret with a few women whom I worried might meet this description. When we have these kinds of fears in the back of our mind at all times, we tend to start seeking relationships following the "safer" gender roles (even if we're not fully aware of it), where the woman acts coy and the man initiates. And once we fall into this dynamic, it becomes so hard to break out of it.

Fortunately, I met Vanessa before I fell too far into that traditional pattern. Even though we had a number of conversations early on about the outdated gender roles that we didn't want in our relationship, I still found something eating away at me whenever I felt like she was initiating sex "too much." Instead of feeling flattered or grateful to have a partner who desired me, I found myself questioning why *I* wasn't initiating sex first. Was I not man enough? Wasn't I supposed to want it more than she did? Was something wrong with my sex drive? And let me tell you, once you start having those thoughts running through your head, you're not gonna feel very sexy. It took a long time for me to recognize what I was putting myself through, and in the meantime, it caused a lot of hurt to both of us. I found myself reacting negatively to Vanessa's initiations (in reality I was just reacting to that voice in my head, but how could she know that?) and beating myself up inside, while causing Vanessa to question whether I wanted her.

We've come to learn that there must be a balance of initiation in every relationship. While those typical gender roles may feel easy and familiar at first, over time they become a trap. When you're the one who never or rarely initiates, sex can start to feel like something your partner always wants from you—which, over time, can come to feel like a burden. Sex can seem like something that happens *to* you rather than something you actively participate in. It can also be hard to tune into your own desire; if your partner is always the one to initiate, you lose the opportunity to discover when you genuinely want sex. On the flip side, when you're the perpetual initiator, you eventually start to wonder if your partner ever actually wants sex, or you may even start to feel resentful that they don't initiate. Even if you're comfortable initiating most of the time, you still want to know that your partner wants you! Because who doesn't want to feel desired?

Using Your Partner's Initiation Style

After some tough love, I've gotten Jacee and Blue on board with stepping out of their comfort zones and initiating with each other more directly.

"I feel stupid asking this question, but how do I do it?" Blue asks. I can tell she's looking at me because she's too embarrassed to look directly at Jacee. "I don't know what's sexy. Is that even the right word?"

"That's a *great* question!" I tell her. "First, initiation should feel like an *invitation*. Think about how you initiate friend dates. You would never call up a friend and say, 'I guess it's been a while. We should probably hang out, huh?' Instead, you might say, 'Hey, do you wanna come over on Friday? We could do drinks and snacks at my place, then go to that new French restaurant. I'd love to see you!'"

Blue's eyes widen. "I don't know if I've ever initiated sex in a way that felt like an invitation. Yikes."

"Most of us haven't," I tell her. "So let's dive into this a little deeper and figure out each of your Initiation Styles."

I developed this model because so many of the couples I worked with were struggling with initiation. As Gary Chapman says in *The Five Love Languages*, we tend to assume that our partner wants the same thing we do. But we all have different things that turn us on in the moment, and unique ways that we like to be invited to have sex. You might be daydreaming about your partner aggressively pushing you up against a wall, but to your partner that might feel demanding or even unsafe.

Based on my work with thousands of people, I've identified six unique Initiation Styles. Your style is your *preferred* initiation technique. You may respond positively to any of the six styles at any given time, but your Initiation Style is the one you're most likely to say "Hell yes!" to the most consistently.

The Initiation Styles model also thinks about desire in a holistic way, and invites you to think about the mental, emotional, physical, relational, and sensory dynamics that get you interested in sex.

If it feels like the Initiation Styles don't perfectly match your needs, that's fine! You can read them to your partner and say, "This describes me really well, except for this part of it. Here's what that's really like for me." Or even, "I'm a combo of these two types, with this piece from the first type and this piece from the second type."

Excite Me

You want to create an element of anticipation around sex. For you, initiation is a slow burn. You want to keep the Sex Drive Simmer going with your partner for days, teasing each other with knowing looks and taunting touch. You like sex to be an open topic of conversation and initiation to be verbal. You might enjoy scheduling sex because it gives you the opportunity to build up desire. You may also appreciate some additional stimulation to get you going in the moment, like reading erotica or talking dirty.

Take Care of Me

You feel the most turned on when your partner is being a caretaker. You may feel so overloaded and exhausted in your day-to-day life that you need relaxation more than seduction. You love it when your partner does chores without being asked or takes over for you in the moment. You have a hard time closing all the tabs in your brain and shifting into sexy mode, so you appreciate when your partner takes over and gives you a few minutes of alone time. This helps you wind down and come home into your own skin. When you're feeling playful, you love a little choreplay. You like watching your partner ham it up with some sensual vacuuming!

Play with Me

You love when your partner appeals to your playful side. The fastest way to get into your pants is to make you laugh! You don't want sex to feel so serious all the time, and your partner definitely does not need to seduce you. You like having inside jokes for initiation, like a song you always play or an emoji you send to each other.

Desire Me

You want your partner to make you feel desirable. Nothing turns you on more than knowing your partner is turned on by you and *needs* you. For others, that strong sense of need may feel overwhelming, but for you it's a huge turn-on. You like spontaneity, too, like that feeling that your partner has to have you *immediately*. You want your partner to give you tons of compliments and help you see how sexy you are. You may like it when your partner gets assertive with you, like grabbing you out of nowhere or pushing you up against a wall.

Connect with Me

For you, sex is all about that emotional connection. You absolutely need to feel emotional intimacy before you feel open to physical intimacy. You want to spend quality time with your partner and feel like your partner is fully there in the moment with you. You need intimate conversation. You can be hyperattuned to touch, easily susceptible to the Bristle Reaction, because you never want to feel pressured to have sex.

Touch Me

You're the rare type that the Boob Honk might actually work for! You love any sort of physical touch. You don't want your partner to verbally initiate with you; you like them to appeal to your body first. You love it when your partner sneaks up behind you and kisses you on the neck or rubs your back. It's not so much about feeling desired by your partner; it's more about them being willing to put the time into awakening your body.

The Initiation Styles don't have to be limiting. If you're interested in something different in the moment, you can use the list of Styles to name what you want. For example, "Babe, I'm in the mood for a little Take Care of Me action right now" or "I'd be open to some Play with Me at any point today!"

After reading these types, do you see how it can be easy for miscues to happen around turn-ons and initiations? If your partner is a Touch Me type, but you're a Take Care of Me, you're likely to get irritated or even offended if they go straight for a hand down the pants.

For Blue and Jacee, the Initiation Styles provide a huge sense of relief. Blue realizes that she's a Connect with Me type. Jacee had been picturing having to seduce Blue with Desire Me–type moves, so this feels a lot more manageable. But for many couples, the Initiation Styles may still feel quite vulnerable. The good news is that you'll know what your partner will respond best to, so the Initiation Styles will set you up for success. And if you're both making an effort to speak each other's language, it will give you the courage to step out of your comfort zones. Remember—sex is a team sport!

The Other Half with Xander: The Lies Movies Tell Us

After reading about these Initiation Styles, you might be feeling some disappointment. Your partner probably prefers a different type of initiation than you do, and let's be real—having to talk about *how* to initiate, and then do it in a way that feels totally foreign to you, seems like a lot of work!

Most people have a vision of sex as something that goes from zero to sixty in a matter of seconds (and, in a way that none of the Initiation Styles describe). You make eye contact with your partner, five seconds later you're ripping off each other's clothes, and a minute after that you're both lying in the afterglow of the best orgasm of your life! After all, that's how it happens in the movies—so why can't it just happen like that in real life?

I'll answer that question with another question: Why can't you go on a round-the-world adventure, complete a semester of university, or find Blackbeard's buried treasure in just two hours? We all know that in real life this stuff takes a lot longer than it does on the screen, so we subconsciously go along with clearly unrealistic things happening (e.g., our heroine walks out of her apartment in Chicago, suitcase in hand, and appears in Hawaii a moment later, no worse for wear). There's even a term for this—suspension of disbelief—which describes how we disregard the impossible in film for the sake of our own entertainment.

So, the next time you see a steamy sex scene in a movie or show, try to remind yourself that they don't have time to show you everything. You're getting a montage of whatever the director decided were the best bits. And more important, remind yourself that real-life sex takes as long as it takes; it can and should include all kinds of time-intensive activities—kissing, slowly removing clothes, finding comfortable positions, foreplay, intercourse, more foreplay, more intercourse, aftercare, and so on.

Let's Do This

Now it's time to have a chat with your partner about your favorite turn-on techniques. There's one ground rule for this conversation: absolutely no shaming each other about any of your turn-ons. You're not responsible for fulfilling all your partner's needs (more on that later), but you do need to be respectful of them. Don't laugh at your partner because their turn-ons seem random, intense, silly, kinky, or even nonsexual.

Here's what to cover:

- What Initiation Style do you resonate with the most, and why?
- What are three specific ways your partner could invite you to be intimate?
- Go back to your Drive and Reverse lists. Are there any dynamics that help you feel turned on in the moment?

Writing Your Sex Menus

Let me ask you a question you've probably never considered before: What, exactly, are you initiating?

For most of us, the basic request behind initiation is "Do you want to have sex with me?" But there are so many different things that we could be initiating! There are dozens of physical activities that we could do, different amounts of time that we could take or effort that we could make, and even unique emotional tones to physical intimacy. And our reaction to the initiation is going to vary based on what's being initiated. For example, if I've had an exhausting day and am not really in the mood, I'm going to have a very different reaction to Xander if he asks me for a quickie versus a night of long, slow, romantic sex.

When all you ask is "Do you want to have sex?" it's sort of like asking someone if they want to go on a trip with you. If you're really excited about travel, you might be an immediate yes, but in most situations, you're going to want to know more details. Where are we going? When do we leave? For how long are we traveling? How much is it going to cost?

So, my suggestion for leveling up your initiation is to write Sex Menus and incorporate them into initiation! What are you inviting your partner to do? You can have single-item Menus (the sexual equivalent of a hamburger) or multi-course extravaganzas. Writing your Menus as a couple can be a really fun bonding exercise. You can come up with cute names for them like "Taco Tuesday" or "Steak and Potatoes" or "Michelin Star Tasting Menu." When you initiate with your partner, you can let them know which specific Menu you're inviting them to try, or you can give them a few different Menus to choose from.

Let's return to our old friend the Stranger. When it comes to desire, you're always going to be a bit of a stranger to yourself and to your partner. You're never going to be able to draft a perfect User Manual that will work every time. Your arousal needs are going to change throughout the course of your life, and they're never going to be foolproof. The nape of my neck is exquisitely sensitive, and nine times out of ten, I'll get turned on if Xander kisses me there. But at that one out of ten times, I recoil. When I'm in a bad mood, I get frustrated, confused, or sad when Xander can't turn me on. When I'm in a good mood, I think of it as just part of being human. When I'm in a *really* good mood, I tell myself that it's my body's way of keeping my attention. If I had a foolproof routine, after all, I'd never take the time to explore my body and discover new or unusual things that it responds to. And wouldn't that be a shame?

Considering Your Partner's Initiation

Here's one of the crazy things about initiation that no one ever talks about: there is an extremely high likelihood that you're *not* going to be wildly turned on in the exact moment that your partner initiates. You're two different people, with unique needs, and it would be too much of a coincidence for you to both be hot and heavy at the same time, on a consistent and ongoing basis. I wouldn't expect Xander to want to take a shower, or go on a walk, or eat a bowl of strawberries at the exact same time I feel the desire to. Why would sex be any different?

Because the Fucking Fairy Tale only shows couples being interested in sex in the exact same moment, a lot of us feel off guard and embarrassed when our partner initiates and we're not immediately interested. Our knee-jerk reaction is to say no without giving ourselves the opportunity to see if we might potentially be interested. Returning to my travel example from earlier, let's say your friend asks you to go on a trip. Would you judge yourself for wanting more details or some time to mull it over? I doubt it! So let's give ourselves a little "let me think about it" space when it comes to sex, too! I walk Jacee and Blue through a few ways to approach what I call the Consideration process.

"The first thing to do when your partner initiates is to remind yourself that your partner is wanting to feel *connected* to you in that moment. They're initiating emotional intimacy as well as physical. You don't want to downplay their request as their just wanting pure physical release."

"I can do that," Jacee says. "I can even remind myself, 'This is Blue being vulnerable.'"

"Great! The next thing you can do is ask yourself, 'Am I open to seeing if I can get turned on?' or, 'Am I open to connecting with my partner right now?' I like using the word 'open' because it makes it clear that you don't need to be turned on right in that moment. You're aiming for possibility, not for outright lust."

"That makes so much sense," Jacee tells me. "Even after all you've taught us about simmering and whatnot, my sex drive still feels really subtle. I can't picture myself getting wildly turned on when Blue initiates, even if she uses my Initiation Style. But being *open* to intimacy . . . that feels different."

"For me, too," chimes in Blue. "Feels like it lowers the bar."

I continue: "Another option, if your partner hasn't done it already, is to ask them what's on the Menu, or see if there's a different Sex Menu you might be more interested in. And then the real heart of the Consideration process is to give yourself more time to feel into their invitation. You don't have to respond right away. You could say something like, 'Give me ten minutes to finish up this email. Once I've got this off my mind, I'll be able to see if I'm up for it.' Or, even more simply, say: 'Can I take a few minutes to consider your invitation?'"

"I'm not sure I love that idea," says Jacee. "If I'm the one initiating, it might leave me feeling like my rejection is getting even more drawn out. I'd feel anxious waiting for her to respond."

"No problem; you don't have to use that technique," I tell her. "What about this instead? 'I'm not sure how I'm feeling. I'm down to start making out (or massaging each other, or whatever sounds good to you) and see where it goes.' If you don't end up getting turned on, you don't have to keep going."

"That's good for our Responsive asses," Blue laughs. "But what if we start kissing and I *don't* get turned on?"

I turn the question right around to Jacee. "What would you prefer: You and Blue have more make-out sessions, and sometimes it just ends there and you're a little disappointed? Or you only have make-out sessions when Blue can guarantee you that she'll want to do more afterward?"

Jacee laughs. "Easy. More make-outs."

"Seriously?" Blue asks. "I can see you getting a little butthurt about it if I don't want to go further."

"I might be disappointed in the moment, for sure," confesses Jacee, "but I can live with that. I like making out with you."

What's Your Responsibility?

If your partner has a higher sex drive, you've probably felt a sense of guilt or pressure to have sex that you didn't personally want to have. And as I'm sure you already know, when you feel obligated to have sex, you're just not going to actively crave it. Pressure and expectation stop desire in its tracks.

But I see a lot of articles online that say you should have sex with your partner, even if you're not in the mood. It brings up a really interesting question: Are you responsible for fulfilling *all* your partner's sexual needs?

Here's my take: I think it's fine to have sex with your partner when you're not in the mood, or to have sex that's more for them than it is for you. (And remember that Responsive sex drive types won't often get mentally into the mood until after physical intimacy has started.) But I think it's extremely important that you (a) recognize that you *always* have a choice when it comes to anything you do with your body, and (b) make the conscious decision to be intimate even though you're not (yet) in the mood. You're *not* agreeing to get naked because you feel guilt or pressure. You're only doing it because it feels safe and good to take care of your partner in that moment, and because they are sometimes willing to have sex that is more for your sake than for theirs. Goodwill and reciprocity are essential for this to work.

At the same time, it's my firm belief that we are not responsible for meeting *all* our partner's sexual needs. Yes, part of being in a relationship is taking care of each other and doing things for each other. But we can never fulfill every single one of our partner's needs at all times, inside the bedroom or outside it. Because if we did, we'd be playing the role of a servant, not a partner.

How to Say No

Whenever I talk about initiation, couples almost always assume I'm going to teach them how to get on board with their partner's requests. But research has shown that being able to say no to sex is critically important. In one study, researchers took a look at how couples handled being turned down for sex. In some relationships, the partner who said no would get punished with the silent treatment, anger, or guilt tripping. In other relationships, the nos were respected. Which group do you think had more sex? The latter![1] So, you really want to make sure that you make it okay to say no in your relationship.

If you're just not open to being intimate with your partner in a given moment, let's go through how to turn your partner down in a way that will bring the two of you closer together instead of pulling you apart.

First, give your partner a specific reason why you're saying no. To be clear, you're always allowed to say no to sex for no reason in particular. It's your body, and you get to decide what you want to do with it. But hearing a specific reason why you're not up for it in that moment can soften the blow for your partner. If they understand that you're stressed out about your upcoming presentation, or worried about your mom's health, they'll be more understanding and less likely to get their feelings hurt.

Here's the key to this step: you also want to talk about how that specific reason impacts your ability to show up for your partner or yourself in the way that you want. So, for example, if you just tell your partner, "I have a headache," that sounds like the most classic and fake-sounding excuse in the book, right? But listen to this instead: "My head is throbbing right now, and I can't focus on anything other than the pain. I really want to be able to be present in the moment with you and be playful like we usually are, but I know I just can't get into that space right now." Sounds so much better, right? Your partner understands that it's not just a lame excuse; it actually impacts the connection the two of you would be able to share. You're essentially telling your partner, "I'm turning down sex right now, for this reason, but I'm not turning down *you*."

Giving a specific reason also presents you with another chance to see if you might actually be open to intimacy. You may get so tense when you know your partner is about to initiate that you might forget to check in with yourself about whether or not you're actually interested in having sex. Thinking of your reason for turning down intimacy gives you a moment to consider whether you could open up to connecting with your partner.

It also helps you understand what's going on for you. Taking the time to discover your real reasons for not wanting to have sex helps you get to know yourself better. There's valuable insight to uncover. For example, you might start to realize that energy plays a big role in your interest in sex. You could tell your partner something like, "By the time we get to the end of the night, I'm just too tired for sex. But if you were to initiate with me when we first get home from work, I might be more game." Or, "I've noticed that I sometimes feel overwhelmed when you initiate sex, and I can tell that you want to be intimate right then and there. I like it when you send me a text during the day telling me that you want to be intimate later. That gives me time to prepare and get excited." The idea is for you and your partner to help set each other up for success by teaching each other the best times and best ways to initiate.

Here's an interesting little wrinkle in this whole issue: if your first reaction is *always* to say no, I've found that it's often a sign you're not saying no to your partner in other areas of your life. That is, your resentment about doing more than your fair share of chores can come spilling out in resistance to sex. Again, you're always allowed to say no to sex, for whatever reason. But if you find yourself having a knee-jerk no instinct even when you're actually a yes, it's an opportunity to get curious about other areas of your life where you may need to say no.

Let's Do This

Talk to your partner about how you can each turn the other down in the gentlest way possible. Here are some questions to ask each other:

"Is there a specific phrase or action I can do to show you that I still love you and am attracted to you, even though I don't feel open to physical intimacy in that moment?"

"How does it feel if I share a genuine reason in the moment?"

"Is there any way you would adjust Vanessa's advice to make it feel better for you?"

Navigating Common Pitfalls

"If I turn my boyfriend down for sex, he pouts, and it feels like a punishment. This makes me feel like I'm not allowed to say no. When I bring it up, he says he's allowed to have his own feelings about it."

It's important that you both make space for disappointment in your relationship. When you say no to your partner, he's probably going to feel embarrassed, hurt, sad, self-conscious, or a combination of the above. Those are understandable feelings that he's allowed to have.

That being said, the word "punishment" feels like a red flag to me. It's not acceptable for him to get angry or attempt to guilt or pressure you into changing your no into a yes.

It can help to identify beforehand a specific phrase that your partner can use in the moment, like, "I'm bummed out that we're not going to connect, but I hear and respect that you're not open to it right now." That gives him the opportunity to express his feelings, but without it coming across as a punishment.

"My partner can't seem to get my Initiation Style right. I told him I'm a Desire Me type, and I want him to be assertive. He tried, but it felt so inauthentic. I haven't given him feedback because I don't want him to feel discouraged. But honestly, it's a turn-off to have to teach a man how to be dominant."

Of course it would be nice if your partner got it right on the first try, but that's just not realistic. If Desire Me isn't his Initiation Style, it's going to take time and repetition for him to home in on what works. And you need to be his patient teacher. You're putting him in an unfair position by being unwilling to help him learn what you want. If verbal instruction doesn't seem to be getting the point across, try *showing* him how you want sex initiated.

If it's still not landing, say something like, "I'm curious to know what it's like for you trying to tap into my style. What does it bring up for you?" I've worked with plenty of men in the past who didn't like being dominant in the bedroom because it felt too caveman-like.

"I tried to talk to my partner about their turn-ons, and they said, 'I could go without ever having sex again and be perfectly fine.'"

Around 1 percent of the population identifies as asexual, and it's possible that your partner is part of that group. However, asexuality is a lifelong disinterest in sex. Many of my clients have said they would be fine never having sex again, but 95 percent of the time it was more a reflection of the pressure and conflict in the relationship than their true sexual identity. They're not saying "I never want to have sex again"; they're saying "I never want to *fight* about sex again."

I suggest trying to get your partner involved in reading *Sex Talks* with you. Say something like, "I know that our sex life has been a source of tension. I want to feel true closeness and intimacy with you. I've been learning a lot of other aspects of sex in this book, and I'd love for you to read it with me. Would you be open to that?"

It may also help to tweak your language. The word "turn-on" can feel too strong for some people. Instead, you can try "When do you feel the most connected to me?" or "What's something I do that makes you feel good?"

"My wife thinks my low sex drive is an issue of attraction. She says, 'I must not be that attractive to you if you're never in the mood.' I am attracted to her, but nothing I say seems to help her anxiety."

It's easy to fall into the trap of thinking desire and attraction are the same thing. But in all my years of doing sex therapy, attraction has rarely been the central problem for a couple. There are dozens of factors that can affect sex drive, and attraction is just one of them.

If you've identified the specific dynamics that are influencing your sex drive, share those with your wife. If many of them are "Me" dynamics, tell her, "My sex drive exists independent of you. This is definitely not what I want, but if you and I were to break up tomorrow, I'd still have many of the same issues I'm having." If you've identified some "We" dynamics, discuss how the two of you can be a team in working on those.

It's also valuable to sympathize with the anxieties coming up for her. Say something like, "It sounds like this brings up a lot of fear for you. I can imagine it feels really scary to wonder if I'm attracted to you or not. If I were in your situation, I would feel that same fear. I want you to know that I absolutely, unequivocally am attracted to you."

I know it's painful to watch your wife struggle with her feelings of desirability, but I also want to remind you that it's not your responsibility to ensure that she feels attractive at all times.

"I want to talk about how I can turn my husband down gently. But in the history of our relationship, I've always been the one doing the turning down. (In comparison, he's probably turned me down once or twice in ten years.) I'm

worried he's going to jump to saying something like, 'Just don't turn me down. That's what would be better,' which of course would prevent us from having a useful conversation about it."

Head your partner off at the pass before initiating this conversation. Say something like, "I know that I'm the one who does the turning down the vast majority of the time, and I can imagine that has been really hard for you. I want there to be less tension in our sex life, so I've been putting a lot of work into better understanding myself. I want us to work as a team to get on the same page." Have a separate conversation about that, before you even get to talking about initiation and consideration.

Once you do talk about turning each other down, remind your partner of the context. Tell him, "While we're working on improving our sexual communication and our overall sex life, there's one specific conversation that I'd like to have with you about how we handle individual moments when I'm truly not open to physical intimacy."

JUST THE TIP(S):

- It's time to share your "Me" sex drive dynamics with your partner.
- The Sex Drive Simmer is a way of creating the potential for desire to arise in the first place.
- It's common and normal in a male-female relationship for the woman to want sex more.
- Initiating sex requires both you and your partner to be vulnerable.
- Your Initiation Styles will teach you the most effective way to invite your partner to be intimate.
- Writing your Sex Menus as a couple can be a sexy and fun bonding experience.
- There is an extremely high likelihood that you're not going to be turned on in the exact moment that your partner initiates. That's what the Consideration process is for.
- In a healthy relationship, you need to be able to turn down sex without repercussions.

Now that we've gotten sex started, it's time to move into making it feel good!

CHAPTER 8

THE FOURTH CONVERSATION:
Pleasure

aka, "What Do We Each Need to Feel Good?"

NOW THAT WE'RE over halfway through the book, you've gotten to know Xander a bit. You probably think he seems like a pretty nice guy, right? Well, let me tell you about how Xander acted like a real dick at the very beginning of our sexual relationship.

When Xander and I met, I was in the midst of a pretty challenging period in my sexual history. I was studying to be a sex therapist, and I was struggling with a serious case of imposter syndrome because I had a big secret: I couldn't orgasm with a partner. I had figured out how to climax on my own, but it wasn't translating to my partnered sexual experiences. So, I did what most women in my situation do: faked orgasms. For years.

Faking seemed like the best solution because the thought of communicating openly about my orgasm problem felt horrifying. I certainly didn't want to open my mouth and tell my partners that I had no clue how to climax with another person. When I started sleeping with someone new, I wanted things to feel effortless and easy, like we were clicking. I also didn't know what the heck I would say even if I could work up the courage to talk. Nothing had made me orgasm in the past, so what was I supposed to tell my partner? "Keep trying!" I also felt a strange duty to protect my partner's ego. I didn't want someone thinking they were "bad in bed" because they couldn't get me there. I was the one who was broken, after all. (Or so I thought . . .)

But as anyone who has ever pretended to have an orgasm knows, faking really sucks. Right before meeting Xander, I had gotten so fed up with years of unsatisfying sex that I decided it was time to finally figure out this whole climax thing. I resolved not to fake it with Xander.

Our relationship started off great. He seemed like a sweet, funny, interesting guy. Like I mentioned in the Intro, the chemistry was definitely there. But after some exciting experiences in the beginning, things just felt . . . off. Intimacy was fun, but he didn't seem to pay much attention to my experience. He would touch me or go down on me for a minute or two (definitely not long enough for me to orgasm), then move on to intercourse. He'd have an orgasm on his own timeline, without trying to help me have one, or even asking me if I was satisfied. I felt so confused. How could this guy seem like such a catch in every other area, but such a selfish jerk in the bedroom?

I had resolved to stop faking orgasm, but I still didn't have the skill set to communicate about it. So, I ended up doing the worst possible thing: waiting until I was bubbling over with resentment, right after we'd just had sex (he was still in the afterglow of his own climax, which triggered me even more), and attacking him about his timing instead of talking about myself and my needs. I don't remember exactly what I said, but it was probably something like, "So, you just do your own thing and then sex is over, huh?"

Credit to Xander that he stayed calm and collected. Launching a grenade the way I did would have led to a massive fight for most couples. Instead, Xander asked me what I wanted from sex. The anger drained right out of me as I realized he was genuinely curious, but I was still sweaty and stammering with awkwardness.

"I don't know," I said. "I guess I just want to feel like you care about me enjoying it, too."

I could see the light bulb go on in his brain, and he launched into an explanation of his previous relationship. Xander's girlfriend before me had struggled with her orgasm, too. But she had told Xander that women don't consistently climax with their partners, that it was fine either way, and that the polite thing for him to do was to focus on himself. This whole time, he had been thinking he was being kind and considerate by not "pressuring" me to have an orgasm with him! As he later put it, "I thought I had the cheat code to female orgasm! I didn't realize I was coming off as a self-centered jerk."

Fortunately, I've since learned how to talk about wants and needs in the bedroom in a much more helpful way. And I now know that I'm not the only one who struggles to talk about what brings us pleasure. My inbox is filled with stories like "I have literally zero clue what to ask for in the bedroom" and "I don't have the heart to tell him he's actually hurting me when he paws at my clitoris like a DJ scratching a record." If you're *lucky*, you've had a partner shyly ask you, "Was it good for you?" but you probably only had the heart to mumble, "Yeah."

There are so many dynamics that make it hard to speak up about what makes us feel good in the bedroom. Pleasure itself is a remarkably challenging concept. I mean, have you ever really taken much time to think about it? How do you define pleasure? What brings you enjoyment and satisfaction? What's the experience of pleasure like for you? If you're like most people, these questions are bewildering.

Most of us think simply of "feeling good." Of course, we can feel pleasure in our bodies, but that's not the whole picture. Pleasure can feel just as fleeting—if not more so—as emotional connection. Xander could stroke my clitoris in the exact same way, but so many different factors will affect the level of enjoyment I feel in a given moment: Are we having angry makeup sex or sweet, slow, romantic sex? Does it seem like he's enjoying himself, or does it seem like he's wishing I would hurry up? Do we have privacy?

Are the lights too bright? Am I thinking about my to-do list? Am I on my period? Pleasure can be physical, but also mental, emotional, situational, energetic, relational, and/or spiritual.

Pleasure isn't fixed, either. Even if I have ideal circumstances in place, my level of enjoyment and satisfaction will still fluctuate in the moment. For me, pleasure feels like waves, with intensity rising and falling in no identifiable cause-and-effect pattern, even if the stimulation stays the same.

Pleasure is too slippery to pin down, even for ourselves. So, how the heck are we supposed to communicate any valuable feedback to our partner?

Even if we *did* know how exactly to describe and ask for pleasure, the Fucking Fairy Tale makes communication feel more complicated. We're taught to believe great sex should just happen "naturally," no communication required. Early in a relationship, we often tell little lies to new partners ("That was so great"; "Yes, I loved that") because we don't want to hurt feelings or because we want to avoid an awkward discussion. But when that new partner turns into a long-term relationship, those fabrications have a way of adding up and tacitly giving us permission to keep lying or withholding.

Plus, our old friend Sexual Perfectionism often comes into play, and we feel pressured to tell our partner exactly what to do (and guarantee that we will like it). And we even have the tendency to believe that once we give our partner a piece of feedback, we're not allowed to change our mind. It's as if we think we get one shot to tell our partner what we like or don't like, and then our answers are locked in for life!

But we need to talk about pleasure in the bedroom, so that you can have an enjoyable experience! This Sex Talk should be your starting point if you're not currently experiencing much pleasure during sex, if you feel like you have no idea what makes sex good for you, or if you've never shared that information with your partner. The conversation will be crucial for you if you feel uncomfortable giving feedback or making requests. And it's an absolute necessity if sex feels one-sided, like there's a noticeable mismatch between the amount of pleasure that you and your partner each experience.

This conversation may also be the key to unlocking your sex drive. Two of the most common reasons for low sex drive are a lack of a connection and a lack of enjoyment. There's a reason why the conversation about desire is bookended by "What Do We Need to Feel Close to Each Other?" and this chapter.

Let's talk about how to have genuinely useful conversations about what feels good to you during sex!

Making Your Touch Maps

Pleasure is a complex topic, so I want to start you off with something simple and straightforward: understanding how you and your partner each like to be touched. On the following pages are some fun exercises for you and your partner to do together. The exercises will help you "map" out each other's bodies. (Important note: these lists aren't set in stone. You're always welcome to revisit and update them!)

"Where I Like to Be Touched"

The following is a list of body parts. Circle all the parts you like to have touched. You can also rate each part from 1 to 5, with 1 meaning "I don't mind being touched here" and 5 meaning "I loooove being touched here." (0 can be reserved for "I don't want to be touched here.")

Toes	Butt	Sides of the neck
Feet	Lower back	Nape of the neck
Ankles	Lower abdomen	Jaw
Calves	Mid-back	Lips
Shins	Chest	Cheeks
Knees	Breasts	Forehead
Behind the knees	Nipples	Scalp
Thighs	Shoulders	Other:
Inner thighs	Front of the neck	

"How I Like to Be Touched"

Next, circle all the *ways* you like to be touched. You can also match specific types of touch with specific parts of the body. For example, "I like to be touched gently on my breasts, and I like to be scratched on my back."

Slowly	Tickled	Massaged
Quickly	Scratched	Spanked
Gently	Pinched	Slapped
Firmly	Hugged	Choked
Squeezed	Spooned	Other:
Caressed	Rubbed	

"Where I Like to Be Kissed"

Again, circle as many as you'd like, or rate from 1 to 5.

Toes	Butt	Sides of the neck
Feet	Lower back	Nape of the neck
Ankles	Lower abdomen	Jaw
Calves	Mid-back	Lips
Shins	Chest	Cheeks
Knees	Breasts	Forehead
Behind the knees	Nipples	Scalp
Thighs	Shoulders	Other:
Inner thighs	Front of the neck	

"How I Like to Be Kissed"

Feel free to match specific kissing styles with specific parts of the body.

Slowly	With shallow tongue contact	With kisses all around the lips
Quickly	With deep tongue contact	With eye contact
Gently	With biting	With no eye contact
Firmly	With breaks between kisses	Other:
With a little bit of tongue		
With a lot of tongue		

"The Energy That Turns Me On"

It can also be really useful to talk about the kind of energy you like to experience with your partner when you're being physically intimate. The following is a list of possible feelings. You may be in the mood for different experiences at different times, but this list can be an interesting conversation starter!

Adventurous	Generous	Romantic
Affectionate	Gentle	Safe
Athletic	Goofy	Sensitive
Careful	Intense	Sensual
Connected	Intimate	Silly
Considerate	Kinky	Slow
Creative	Lively	Spiritual
Edgy	Loving	Surprising
Emotional	Naughty	Sweet
Energetic	Nurturing	Thoughtful
Exciting	Open-minded	Vulnerable
Experimental	Passionate	Warm
Expressive	Playful	Wild
Focused	Rejuvenating	Other:
Fun	Relaxed	

Your Sex Personality Type

Next, I want to give you a framework for getting to know what brings you pleasure—it's your Sex Personality Type. It's not the whole picture, but it will show you the lens through which you filter your experience of sex. In my work with thousands of clients, I came to realize that we all experience enjoyment in unique ways, and we need different circumstances in place in order to enjoy physical intimacy. By identifying which one of the eleven Sex Personality Types you resonate with the most, you'll learn valuable information about how you define and experience pleasure. (You'll likely relate to more than one type, but try to pick the one that most closely defines you.)

You'll also notice that the Sex Personality Types fall into one of three categories:

- Body
- Mind
- Spirit

As I mentioned in the Intro, pleasure can be experienced in myriad ways, but I've found that these are the three most common categories. You can experience enjoyment in all three places, but you'll likely have a primary locus of pleasure. Or you may need to have one type stimulated first, before you can unlock pleasure in other ways. Body-based types are deeply in tune with pure physical sensation. Mind-based types need to feel mentally and intellectually stimulated. Spirit-based types are all about the energy, emotion, and intimacy of sex.

The Decompressor (Body)

For you, sex is all about stress relief. You get enjoyment out of the act itself, but your primary source of pleasure comes at the end, when you've had a release. You love nothing more than basking in the afterglow when sex is over. Physical intimacy is a way that you blow off steam and unwind, and you typically seek it out when you're feeling tense. You may masturbate for the same reasons, too. Orgasms are important to you because they bring about that feeling of relief or release. Sex just doesn't feel complete without that.

The Explorer (Mind)

Sex is your playground! For you, pleasure is all about novelty. You're curious about sex, and you get genuine enjoyment from learning, experimenting, and trying new things. You like pushing yourself out of your comfort zone. In that way, a number of different acts can bring you pleasure; you don't have or want a set routine. You don't take sex too seriously, and you can laugh about it if your explorations don't work out perfectly. You may read articles or books about sex, so it's no surprise that you picked up *Sex Talks* in the first place!

The Fair-Trader (Mind)

For you, equality is the most important aspect of sex. In order for you to feel pleasure, there needs to be a balance between you and your partner of giving and receiving. It's important to you that you and your partner are both enthusiastic. You like knowing that you're both open to each other's needs and are willing to work together to make sure everyone who wants an orgasm gets an orgasm. This can sometimes make feeling pleasure in the moment tricky for you, since you're so fixated on the equilibrium that you can sometimes tune out your own experience.

The Giver (Mind)

You view sex and pleasure as a gift that you give to your partner. Your partner's sexual experience is at least as important to you as your own, but typically even more so. You're very in tune with your partner's experience, and it makes you feel good to know that you can make your partner feel good. You tend to struggle with receiving pleasure, and it's challenging for you to pay attention to your own body in the moment.

The Guardian (Spirit)

For you, it's extremely important for sex to feel safe, and you're not able to feel pleasure unless it does. You need that foundation of security with your partner and with yourself. Your boundaries are important to you, as is enthusiastic consent. You may have experienced sexual abuse in your past, which has led you to seek out safety as an adult. Prior negative experiences with sex may make tuning into your own body feel trickier. Or you may simply like feeling that bond of trust and security with a partner before and while being intimate.

The Passion-Pursuer (Spirit)

You get the most pleasure when sex feels all-encompassing, intense, and passionate. Maybe even animalistic. You're very in tune with the energy between you and your partner during sex, and that energy is even more important than the physical sensations. You love the idea of letting go and losing yourself in the moment. In your opinion, the best sex is when time seems to stand still.

The Pleasure-Seeker (Body)

For you, sex is about pure physical pleasure. You just like to feel good! You may even be confused about all these different personality types, because you think sex is just one of those simple pleasures in life. You enjoy touch and physical contact throughout the day, too. You don't need to feel emotional connection with someone to have great sex with them. You may be a kinesthetic type of person—you learn by doing, and you're tactile.

The Prioritizer (Mind)

The most important thing for you is that sex is something you and your partner prioritize over other things in your life. You don't want to make excuses about being too busy or tired; you want to be intimate before that. You value your sex life, and you're willing to spend time on it and make sacrifices for it. You like sex to be consistent, and you may even like having a specific routine for how often you have sex. For you, pleasure is all about the circumstances. You enjoy yourself the most when the scene has been set, and there's enough time and privacy to focus on each other.

The Romantic (Spirit)

Sex is all about connection for you. You want to experience real emotional intimacy with your partner while you're being physical. It's important for both you and your partner to feel present in the moment with each other. Sometimes you may like slower, more drawn-out experiences. You like exchanging "I love yous" during sex or making eye contact. Pleasure is much more about the intimacy between you and your partner than the pure physical act.

The Spiritualist (Spirit)

You enjoy sex that connects you to a higher purpose, and you think it should be a transcendent experience. Pleasure is so much bigger than what's happening in the body. You may be religious, or you may enjoy Eastern philosophies like Tantra.

The Thrill-Seeker (Mind)

For you, there's a thrill to having sex that feels forbidden or taboo. You may enjoy an element of power play in your sex life, like allowing your partner to dominate you, or your dominating your partner. Whereas the Explorer simply likes exploration for exploration's sake, your pleasure is all about the taboo.

———

I teach the Sex Personality Types to Bella and Soraya, a mixed-orientation couple who started sex therapy because Bella can't consistently orgasm with Soraya. (Bella is bisexual, Soraya is a lesbian.) Soraya feels a deep sense of shame about this. "I'm a cis woman; I have the same parts. I like to think that I know what I'm doing. Why can't I get her there?"

Together, we discover that Soraya is a Pleasure-Seeker, so she's focused on body-based pleasure. (I had a hunch after her comment "I have the same parts.") But Bella is a Romantic, and when Soraya gets fixated on technique rather than on their emotional connection, Bella feels lonely. The discovery of their Sex Personality Types is a relief to Soraya, because she was feeling so much anxiety about her sexual performance.

I help Bella uncover, and then teach Soraya, the specific ways to tune in to her Romantic. A few weeks later, they report back that this approach is working wonders for them. Soraya sets the mood by lighting candles, putting on music, and drawing a bath for the two of them. They make eye contact and talk about how much they love each other. Bella finds herself able to orgasm quickly with Soraya focusing more on purring sweet nothings into her ear than on doing complicated maneuvers with her fingertips.

Let's Do This

Ask each other the following questions:

"Which Sex Personality Type(s) do you resonate with the most, and why?"
"Are you a body, mind, or spirit type?"
"What have you learned about the way you experience pleasure?"

No matter how familiar you get with your unique way of experiencing pleasure, you're never going to reach the point where you're able to accurately predict exactly what you need in a given sexual interaction. Remember that pleasure is too amorphous for us to pin down in this way.

Instead, your primary communication task for the Pleasure conversation is going to be to stay in tune with your own experience in the moment (remember the PLEASE acronym from Part One, and I'll share another exercise later in this chapter) and share it with your partner.

Finding Pleasure through Feedback

I know, I know, you're already starting to sweat, thinking about giving your partner feedback in the bedroom. That's probably because you're still thinking that feedback equals criticism. But feedback is simply reporting back on your experience. In Conversation 1, we started with talking about sex after the fact in a positive way, and we're going to continue that theme by focusing on getting comfortable talking about what happens *during* sex.

First, let's talk about why we even need feedback in the first place. It's hard for a lot of us to wrap our heads around that. I'm constantly inundated with messages like, "My partner can't possibly think I like that, can they?" and, "We've been together for years now; shouldn't my partner just know what to do?" But feedback is a necessary part of any healthy and happy sex life! It's just plain unfair to expect your partner to read your mind at *any* time, but especially when it comes to something as personal as what brings you pleasure. And remember that you've probably given your partner a lot of false or misleading feedback—all those little lies we discussed earlier.

If you're still not convinced, let me ask you this: How is your partner supposed to know what you enjoy most during sex, or whether you're enjoying it at all? Do you do or say anything specific to ensure they know you're having a good time? If you're thinking, "Well, my partner can probably sense what's going on in the moment," then I have another question for you: Does your partner do a fantastic job of reading your mind *outside* the bedroom?

Ryan, a member of our Instagram community, wrote to us: "My fiancée is silent in bed. No words, no moaning, no heavy breathing, no nothing. It's always tough for me to know if she's enjoying herself. Sometimes I think I can tell because she gets a sudden burst of moisture." Think about that. This man is so lost about his partner's experience that he's relying on "a sudden burst of moisture" to indicate to him that she's enjoying herself. And worse—remember our old friend nonconcordance? (It describes the disconnect between our physiological arousal and our mental desire.) Wetness is *not* an indicator of how turned on a vulva is. This guy's one and only sign that his fiancée is enjoying herself isn't even accurate!

Feedback is necessary because, without it, we're also subject to some serious miscommunications. That's exactly what happened to Xander and me once we overcame our initial orgasm hurdles and I started having them regularly. I'm typically a pretty, let's say, vocal person in the bedroom! But the way my orgasm works is that the closer I get, the quieter and stiller I get. I tune in to the building waves of pleasure and focus on what that pleasure feels like rippling throughout my body. But from Xander's perspective, he would see me go from moaning and writhing around on the bed to all of a sudden being silent and stationary, and he felt like he was doing something wrong. So, he would change his technique, trying to find something that would work better. But that would send me back a few steps with my orgasm, prolonging the whole process! Even the tiniest bit of feedback about where I was in my orgasmic journey would have saved us both a lot of hassle.

Feedback is especially important for survivors of sexual abuse. Certain acts, positions, or words can evoke discomfort in the moment or even trigger memories of the abuse. It's essential for survivors to be able to communicate with their partner before, during, and after sex in order to create as much safety as possible.

The bottom line is this: even if it seems painfully obvious to you, you still need to tell your partner what you want. Screw the Fucking Fairy Tale; your partner doesn't know you better than you know yourself, and they don't have a crystal ball to consult that will tell them what to do next.

The good news about feedback is that you don't have to hand over a set of detailed, step-by-step instructions about exactly what to do to you and when. Instead, feedback is all about reporting back to your partner about your experience, in the moment, moment by moment. Feedback can be as simple as "That feels good" or "Don't stop." It doesn't need to be a ten-page manifesto.

It may also bring you some peace of mind to know that you don't need to know you'll like something in order to ask for it. When you go to a restaurant and order the grilled chicken, are you telling the waiter "I solemnly swear that I will *love* this chicken more than I have ever loved any chicken"? Of course not! You're curious about the chicken and you have a pretty good sense that you'll like it, but you won't know until you actually take a bite. A request is not a promise; it's just a request.

Now, a lot of people hear the phrase "giving feedback" and picture themselves telling their partner "You suck at talking dirty" or "Your kissing technique is terrible!" Of course, if you say something like that, it's going to bruise your partner's ego. But that's not the only way to share your experience with your partner! Instead, let me teach you a better way.

Positively Pleasurable Feedback

When you first start communicating about pleasure in the bedroom, focus on grounding all your comments in something positive. Ask for more of what feels *good* instead of criticizing what feels *bad*. This is going to feel easier for you to give, and easier for your partner to receive.

So, you want to avoid saying things like:

"That doesn't feel good."
"No, not like that."
"Don't touch me there."

And instead aim for things like:

"When you touch me here, it feels amazing."
"I like when you use that level of pressure."
"That feels even better than what you were doing before."
"That slower stroke you were doing a minute ago felt great."

(A quick caveat: if you ever experience physical or emotional discomfort or pain, be more direct with your partner and tell them you need to stop. No one should ever experience pain during sex, and I don't want you prolonging that experience because you're trying not to hurt your partner's feelings.)

Positively Pleasurable Feedback works so well, for a number of different reasons. First, it's genuinely useful. Sexual communication is so rare that most people have no clue if what they're doing is working. Positively Pleasurable Feedback gives us the coaching we need and deserve.

Second, it's a lot of fun to get a compliment. It makes your partner feel proud, which will only motivate them to want to keep doing more.

Third, it's really sexy in practice. It can be a huge turn-on for your partner to hear you talk about how good you're feeling and what you like. What sounds better? "You need to put your fingers inside when you go down on me" or "It's so hot when you go down on me. You know what would make it feel even more incredible? If you put two fingers inside of me while you licked my clit. I'm getting excited just thinking about that!" When I share Positively Pleasurable Feedback with my clients, it feels so doable and sexy that they can't believe they felt so self-conscious about giving feedback in the first place.

You can even use Positively Pleasurable Feedback as a sneaky way to make a request. If there's something you'd like your partner to do more frequently, give them a preemptive compliment outside of the bedroom or in the lead-up to intimacy. For example, "Do you know how hot you look when you're going down on me?" or "I can't believe how good you make me feel when you go slow." You're pumping up your partner with confidence and getting them excited to fulfill your request. They very well may catch on and respond with something like, "Is that you asking me for a blow job?" But you can laugh and say, "I guess I am! You're just so good at it!"

Positively Pleasurable Feedback is specifically focused on body-based pleasure, because I've found that to be the easiest starting place for most people. Once you get comfortable tuning in to your physical experience and being more vocal, you can give Positively Pleasurable Feedback about mind-based ("It turns me on to read *Sex Talks* with you") and spirit-based ("I can feel you being fully present with me right now, and I love it") pleasure, too.

Still feeling nervous about actually opening your mouth and talking during sex? Here's a fun exercise you can try: Go back and forth with each other while you're clothed, saying random bits of feedback to each other. They don't have to be things you actually want or like; the idea is just to get comfortable talking. (This is similar to the exercise with Rowena that I shared in the Acknowledgment conversation.) Try saying things like "That feels good," "Keep going," "Can I get on top?" and "Touch my butt." This practice will help you feel more comfortable speaking up in the bedroom, too!

When Lowering Your Expectations Can Actually Be a Good Thing

As you give small bits of feedback to your partner, it's important to be prepared for the possibility that the stimulation you'll receive may not feel that much better than whatever your partner was doing previously. That's because you'll probably be feeling vulnerable or sensitive about the fact that you put yourself out there and started communicating (at least at first)! For example, let's say your partner is giving you a hand job, and you ask them to squeeze a little harder. You're not going to feel fireworks the second they start using a bit more pressure! It might feel 10 percent better than the softer grip your partner had been using a minute earlier. Maybe 1 percent. Or maybe asking for more pressure made your anxiety levels skyrocket for a few seconds, and you're actually feeling even *less* pleasure than you were before!

That's why I encourage you to temporarily lower your expectations and have some patience while you develop a better sense of what feels good for you. As you get more comfortable giving feedback, making requests, and trying new things, aim for small improvements. If it feels just a tiny bit better than what you were doing previously, that's perfectly okay! In the long term, all these smaller improvements in pleasure will compound into far more enjoyable sex overall.

What If My Partner Doesn't Listen?

Margaret, a member of our Instagram community, wrote in to complain that her husband hadn't acted on her requests. "I've told him several times that I want him to take control more often, but he hasn't. I'm hurt that it doesn't seem too important to him." Listen, it would be *amazing* to give your partner a piece of feedback exactly one time and then watch them adhere to your request for the rest of eternity. (The pure ecstasy I would feel if I never had to remind Xander to take out the trash ever again . . .) But that's just not how human behavior works—in or out of the bedroom. Ever tried to get yourself to make a personal change? Even if it was something you were excited about and committed to, you *know* it takes more than one internal pep talk to get consistent results!

Instead, you're going to have to get used to making multiple requests. This sucks, I know! But your desires are worthy of your advocacy. And your partner is worthy of some grace while they get confident about your asks and learn how to follow through.

If general requests aren't working, make them more specific. I instructed Margaret to tell her husband in the morning that she'd be really turned on if he took control that evening, or to ask him right before they started getting intimate. Also, make sure to be clear and specific about what you want. In Margaret's case, "take control" may be so broad that her husband doesn't know what, exactly, to do.

When You Have Tough Feedback to Give

Sometimes there's just no way to put a positive spin on what's going down in the bedroom. Remember Aaliyah and Sebastian, the couple in the open relationship mentioned in Chapter 2? Sebastian liked calling her a "bad girl" during sex, and she hated it. But she also didn't want him to feel embarrassed or ashamed for using the phrase.

I told Aaliyah to talk to Sebastian outside of the bedroom, well after they'd had sex and when he was in a good mood, and say, "I want us to feel comfortable talking about sex and sharing our experiences with each other, even though I know it can feel sensitive sometimes. I've been noticing lately that I'm just not loving the phrase 'bad girl', but I *would* find it sexy if you described how good I was making you feel instead." This framework accomplishes a lot in just a few sentences:

- Stating your positive intentions.
- Reminding your partner that you're on the same team.
- Being gentle but clear about what you *don't* want.
- Providing your partner with an alternate behavior that you *would* enjoy.

Notice that in this example, there's no complaining or whining. That's because you're so much more likely to get your needs met if you make a direct request. Most of us are so uncomfortable with communication that we don't say anything until our frustration bubbles over. (Be brutally honest with yourself—do you more frequently give your partner complaints or requests?) But here's the thing—no one responds well to complaints. When someone tells you they're disappointed, it only serves to bring up shame, not motivation. And worse, you feel stuck because even if you were to change your behavior, you couldn't do anything to erase their initial disappointment.

The Other Half with Xander: Don't Make It About Your Ego

Receiving feedback can be hard! Especially when it's about something we don't feel comfortable discussing or an area we don't feel especially confident in (e.g., sex). This can come up for anyone, but there's a particularly common dynamic that tends to arise with men: the "OMG, my manhood is under attack!" reaction. Remember that embarrassing story Vanessa told at the beginning of this chapter, about how I was only paying attention to my own pleasure during sex? Vanessa was quite generous in her description of how I handled it, because honestly it was hard to hear in the moment, and it took a couple months for me to come to grips internally with how we needed to address the problem. Even though I knew she wasn't having consistent orgasms, I felt like my own sexual prowess was being called into question. It felt like my job as a man—to know what he's doing in bed and to provide—was somehow being threatened.

Those of us who identify with the masculine tend to be socialized to value self-sufficiency and providing for our partner. When it comes to sex, what we see on TV depicts men being assertive and magically pleasing their partners, without those partners ever giving any direction or feedback. Add on the fact that most of us have had past sexual partners who faked orgasm or gave misleading sexual compliments, and you have the perfect storm: someone who desperately wants to provide in the bedroom and mistakenly *thinks* they know exactly what they're doing! So, when we receive an unexpected piece of feedback that challenges this worldview, it's easy to get upset and try to make it about our ego rather than actually listening to the feedback and using it as an opportunity to improve our partner's experience.

With that context in mind, here are a few suggestions for how to deal with this dynamic, regardless of your gender.

If your ego is feeling bruised:

- Trust that your partner has positive intentions with their feedback. Of course, we all want to feel like we're incredible in bed, and it's hard to hear even the tiniest hint that we're not perfect sexual mind readers. But trust that your partner has the best of intentions with what they're sharing. They're not trying to hurt your feelings; they're being honest in the hope that it brings the two of you closer together and creates a better experience for you both.
- When you deflect by turning feedback into a referendum on your ego, you're effectively burying your head in the sand. You could either

sulk in the knowledge that you're going to keep doing something in bed that your partner doesn't particularly enjoy, or you could take some action and bring them more pleasure. Which of those will feel better to your ego in the long run? (Let's hope the latter . . .)

- Think about how you would prefer to receive feedback. Maybe you'd like a warning before the conversation begins so you can get into the right frame of mind, or you'd prefer it be done via text so you have time to consider your responses. Communicate this to your partner.

If your partner is the one with the bruised ego:

- It's not your job to keep your partner's ego permanently inflated.
- Remind your partner that everyone's body works differently, so your feedback has nothing to do with them "doing something wrong"; in fact, the thing you're giving feedback about may very well have been heaven on earth for a past partner.
- When giving feedback, try to emphasize whatever it is you would like done differently and how pleasurable that will be for *you*, rather than overly focusing on the action your partner is taking and how it's adversely impacting you. For example, "Could you rub my clit gently? It feels so good, and I think I could come pretty fast that way!" versus "Softer! You're ruining my orgasm by rubbing so hard."

The Other Side of the Equation: Asking for Feedback from Your Partner

What if you're the one who wants to know more about your partner's experience in the bedroom? Most of us will ask the question, "What do you want?" But this is one of the *worst* questions to ask in the bedroom because it's too general and it puts your partner on the spot. It's like that classic

"What are we going to have for dinner?" conundrum. If your partner asks you that question, you're going to respond, "I don't know; what do you want?" Then they're going to respond, "I don't know; I asked you first." And on and on. But if they say, "Hey, so I was thinking about dinner tonight. How do you feel about Italian or Chinese?" Now all of a sudden you're considering only two variables instead of an infinite number. Even if you actually want Mexican, the decision still feels clearer and easier to make!

One of the simplest things you can do to improve your sex life is to eliminate the "What do you want?" question from your vocabulary and substitute my Eye Exam Test.

When you go to get your eyes checked out, the optometrist doesn't just sit you down and say, "Describe what you want your vision to be like." Instead, they show you a series of slides and ask you, "Which one is more in focus—one or two?" Sometimes those slides get pretty damned tricky, but in general, choosing between the two options feels straightforward.

You can use the same technique in the bedroom! Give your partner options to choose from, instead of asking them to come up with an answer out of thin air to "What do you want?" For example, "Do you want me to massage your back or your shoulders?" or "Does it feel good when I touch you like this or like *this*?" or "Do you like it better when I use this pressure or *this* pressure?"

The Eye Exam Test also helps your partner feel like you're genuinely invested in bringing them pleasure, because you've taken the time to think of a few specific options. Honestly, "What do you want?" is a lazy question. It's not that hard to come up with a few specific options instead.

Closing the Orgasm Gap

Giving and receiving feedback can make a big difference in the bedroom, but it can't solve the enormous issue of misinformation about female pleasure.

Buckle up, because it's time to talk about one of my favorite topics: equity in the bedroom. I typically see this come up only with cis male-female couplings, so I'm going to focus on that particular gender configuration here.

In 2009, the National Survey of Sexual Health and Behavior asked almost two thousand US-based adults about their most recent sexual experience.[1] The vast majority of these experiences were with a partner of the opposite sex, so this is some pretty heteronormative research. So, 91 percent of men said they climaxed during their last sexual encounter, compared to only 64 percent of women. But a shocking 85 percent of men *thought* that their female partner had orgasmed (that's a 21 percent difference in perception versus reality, in case you're as bad at math as men apparently are at recognizing female pleasure).

Let me give you a glimpse into my email inbox, and share three messages that came in, all in the span of a few hours:

> "My husband says he doesn't feel like taking the time to make sure I orgasm 75 percent of the time. I brought it up again last week and said, 'I just want to have the same experience as you, at least most of the time,' and his response was, 'But it's not the same experience. My orgasm only takes me a few minutes if I want it to. Yours takes way more effort.'"

> "My boyfriend won't go down on me, even though that's the only way I orgasm, because he says he doesn't enjoy doing it. He's given me every excuse: he'll do it some other time, it hurts his neck, I 'taste different,' he has a short tongue that gets tired easily. Side question: Is this tongue issue even a thing?"

> "When my husband and I have sex, it feels very one-sided. He reaches his climax, and then he stops and leaves me hanging. He doesn't mean to be rude; I think he just thinks of his orgasm as the end of sex. Like, 'Okay, I've been satisfied, now I'm done, and therefore we're done.' It upsets me because I want to feel pleasure just as much as he does and have my own orgasm. Am I selfish for thinking this way?"

Let's read that last sentence again: "Am I selfish for thinking this way?" That question boggles my mind. No! It's not selfish to want the same pleasure and satisfaction as your partner is getting. It's not selfish to want the same experience your partner is having.

But the problem is not just that we have a plague of selfish men. A lot of women also struggle to receive pleasure in the bedroom. My friend Francesca tells me, "Jake wants to have a ton of foreplay and spend all this time on sex. It's fun every once in a while, but more often than not, I feel uncomfortable when he tries to focus on me. It takes too much to get me there, and sometimes it doesn't feel worth it. I just want him to have his orgasm and get it over with." Francesca already knows that having "get it over with" sex is soul-sucking (and she realizes the irony of feeling resentful of Jake for the times he brings sex to a close right after getting his). It's never going to feel good for her, she's never going to crave it, and it's certainly not going to lead to any true intimacy between her and Jake. But she's still settling for these scraps because she doesn't feel worthy of more.

I ask Francesca why her non-faked orgasms are few and far between, and she tells me that Jake is too rough with her clitoris. He has used this technique since the beginning of their relationship, and she had faked orgasms for the same reason I did: because it just felt easier. But now it's been years, and she doesn't want to make Jake feel bad by speaking up and telling him it's not working. It's another classic issue that I see: we women are socialized to be hypersensitive to other people's feelings, and to sacrifice our own comfort to preserve a partner's ego.

Why are so many couples struggling to create pleasure equity in the bedroom? As always, it comes back to misinformation and lack of education. We're taught to believe so much BS about female pleasure and orgasm:

- That it's complicated or mysterious.
- That all you need to do as a woman is "just relax" or "just let go and stop thinking about it."

- That you should orgasm from penetration alone and shouldn't require anything "extra" to get there.
- That something must be horribly wrong with you if you haven't had one yet.

Bo and his wife, Elyse, are perfect examples of how this misinformation can be so destructive. They're high-school sweethearts who were virgins when they got married. Bo had been frustrated by how infrequently they had sex, and he thought Elyse's low sex drive was to blame. But then he read an article I wrote about female orgasm, and he realized their mistake.

In our first session, he tells me: "And as far as Elyse and I knew, sex was penis-in-vagina intercourse. For the first seven years, there was nothing in it for her and she hated it, but she felt like she had to have sex on a weekly or twice-weekly basis to meet my needs. Neither of us understood what we were doing wrong, and Elyse thought she was broken because the sex we were having worked fine for me." Elyse suffered in silence for *seven years* because she didn't have basic information about how her body works and what it needs.

Most heterosexual couples are having sex like Bo and Elyse: a few seconds of foreplay, then straight to the intercourse. But penetration is not the most pleasurable activity for the vast majority of women. We polled our Instagram audience, and a whopping 90 percent of women said they prefer something other than intercourse! Our pleasure comes from clitoral stimulation, and we don't get much of that during the ol' P-in-V.

So, let's talk about the clitoris! It's the only part of the human body that exists solely for pleasure. It contains eight thousand to nine thousand nerve endings, whereas the penis contains two thousand to three thousand. But during intercourse, a cis woman is getting stimulation in her vagina, which doesn't have many nerve endings at all. (The ones it does have are located in the outer third of the vagina, so there's even less sensitivity deep inside.)

And did you know that the clitoris and the penis are actually pretty similar? The tissues that make the penis for someone born male are the exact same tissues as make the clitoris for someone born female. So, why do we make women feel bad for needing clitoral stimulation? Because let's get real: whenever you hear the clitoris talked about, it's always something like, "Why do women need this extra stimulation? Why is the clitoris so complicated? It's so hard to find. Does it even exist?" But we don't make men feel bad for needing penile stimulation, right?

From a nerve-ending perspective, intercourse for a woman is the equivalent of a man having his testicles played with. I'm sure there's some very lucky man out there who can orgasm from that, but for most men, it's not gonna happen that way. But let's imagine some alternate universe where what we define as heterosexual "sex" is a man rubbing his testicles on a woman's clitoris. She's getting stimulation on the part of her body that feels the most sensitive. The man might be feeling some pleasure, since the testicles are part of his genitals and do have nerve endings. But would we expect that men would love this new version of intercourse, and that it should be the default sexual activity? Would we make men feel guilty for not getting pleasure from rubbing their testicles on a woman's body? Absolutely not!

I know that sounds like a silly example, but it's *exactly* the situation with penetration. We make women feel terrible for not loving a physical activity that just doesn't stimulate the most sensitive part of their bodies. How shitty is that?

If you're in a male-female relationship and are struggling with an Orgasm Gap, read this section of the book over and over again until you realize there's nothing wrong with you. Then follow our three mantras for pleasure equality in the bedroom:

1: ANYONE WHO WANTS AN ORGASM GETS AN ORGASM
What brings us pleasure is going to look different, but we should all be having enjoyable experiences. A few important caveats, though. The key word is "want." Not everyone wants an orgasm every time, and that's okay. But if someone wants one, you need to work together as a team to make it hap-

pen. Also, orgasm isn't the only way to measure enjoyment and satisfaction. Orgasms are amazing, but try to keep your focus on pleasure itself. After all, you can experience pleasure throughout an entire sexual interaction, but orgasms typically come at the end.

2: REMEMBER YOUR ABCS

If one of you is a vulva owner, make sure to prioritize clitoral pleasure as much as you prioritize penile pleasure. Our rule is ABC: Always Be (touching the) Clit!

3: EVERYTHING COUNTS AS SEX

Do away with the idea that intercourse is the only way to have sex, and put more options on the table. Foreplay can and should be the main event. The same 2009 study by the National Survey of Sexual Health and Behavior that I referenced earlier found that 90 percent of men would orgasm during sex regardless of what sexual activities the couple participated in. But for women, adding more options to the menu greatly increased their likelihood of orgasm. Eighty-one percent could orgasm from oral sex, and 89 percent could orgasm if they engaged in five or more different sexual activities in one interaction. More variety leads to more orgasms!

Don't forget about other forms of pleasure, either. I've focused on body-based pleasure, since the vast majority of people don't know the basic reality of how the clitoris works. But remember that your partner may need mind- or spirit-based forms of pleasure, too.

Let's Do This

Whenever I share the Orgasm Gap with couples, it opens up a lot of conversations. It tends to give couples the ability to "reset" and reconsider so many aspects of their sex life. Here are some questions to discuss:

"How would you like to start exploring clitoral stimulation?"

"What are some things you like to do in the bedroom with me, no matter how big or small they may seem?"

"How can I help you know that I'm on your team in having an orgasm?"

"Are there times when you *don't* want to have an orgasm?"

Navigating Common Pitfalls

"I'll admit that I've done a bad job in the past listening to my wife's feedback, but now she's at the point where she doesn't want to give it to me anymore. She says, 'I've told you what I like already. You should know what to do.'"

It's great that you're taking ownership of past mistakes. Have you shared that with her yet? That could be a great way to open up the conversation. Say something like, "I want to acknowledge that I haven't done a good job listening to your feedback in the past." Share any specific reasons why that was the case for you, like "I felt so insecure about being bad in bed, and it just felt easier to ignore you so I could protect my ego." Continue with something along the lines of, "I'm really sorry for that, and I want things to be different for us going forward. I promise that I'll take your feedback to heart and do my very best to quickly put it into practice."

I also want to remind you and your wife that feedback isn't a one-and-done type of thing! Her preferences may change from moment to moment, experience to experience, and year to year. You can say something like, "I'm also learning to have a different approach to feedback. I want us to be able to communicate about what brings us pleasure for the rest of our lives. I want to learn what you like right now, *and* I also want to make space for what you like to change in the future. Does that make sense to you?"

"I've never had an orgasm with my husband of nine years. I've faked since the beginning. Do I have to come clean?"

I've faked hundreds of orgasms myself, so I get it. But this is why I highly recommend not faking to begin with; you don't want to get into this pickle years down the road!

My recommendation is to come clean and tell your partner. The most important thing for you to recognize is that you didn't fake for malicious reasons. You probably faked because you felt like you were broken and you didn't want your partner to feel broken, too. Tell your partner that! Say something like, "I never, ever wanted to hurt you. I just felt so hopeless that I would ever be able to orgasm, so faking it felt like the best option for us both. I'm really sorry now that I did it, because I can see that I caused a lot of pain for both of us." Your partner is probably going to be surprised and hurt, and may need a bit of time to process their feelings. But this approach does set you up for the greatest chance for orgasmic success moving forward.

If that feels too intimidating, you can try a half-truth approach. Tell your partner that you're noticing that your body is responding to different types of stimulation lately. You can say something like, "I don't know what's going on, but I think I want us to explore a bit more together." That will create more space for the two of you to try different kinds of stimulation.

"My husband and I have some major cultural differences to overcome. His culture believes that vulvas and vaginas are not naturally clean. There's so much shame around sex and fear of germs, so one must be clean to do the deed. Once we started talking about sex, he kept asking me about showering, both before and after sex. I could sense how hard it was for him to not feel all the cultural programming around dirty vulvas, and that made me feel so ashamed of my body."

I didn't have the space in *Sex Talks* to discuss all the unique cultural issues that can come into play with sex, which is really a shame, because there are so many dynamics that can come up, especially when you're talking about different combinations of cultures.

It's completely understandable that your husband has some trepidation about cleanliness after a lifetime of being taught that sex is dirty. However, he now needs to make a choice. Does he want to allow this cultural conditioning to continue affecting his relationship with sex? Or is he ready to move past it? The good news here is that you can probably relate to the negative impacts of cultural conditioning. You can open up a conversation by saying something like, "I understand how your culture has led to these feelings of sex being unclean. I have my own struggles with things I've been taught. I want us both to decide how we *want* to feel about sex moving forward and put effort into changing our relationships with sex. Can you be my teammate in this?"

Working through some of the exercises in Part One of *Sex Talks* can help immensely, as can personal therapy.

JUST THE TIP(S):
- Your Sex Personality Type will give you the lens through which you filter pleasure, including whether you're body, mind, or spirit focused.
- Feedback in the bedroom is crucial. You deserve to ask for what you want, and you don't need to know you'll like something in order to ask for it. The Positively Pleasurable Feedback framework is the best way to do it.
- Use the Eye Exam Test to get helpful feedback from your partner.
- Clitoral stimulation is the key to closing the Orgasm Gap.

Like I mentioned before, pleasure is always in motion. You're never going to be able to fully predict what your body will respond to, nor comprehend exactly what you need. But I hope this chapter has given you tools to stay in the moment and ride the wave with your partner.

Let's wrap up our tour through the Big Five Conversations with the final frontier: exploring what *comes* next. (Pun obviously intended!)

CHAPTER 9

THE FIFTH CONVERSATION:
Exploration

aka, "What Should We Try Next?"

WHENEVER PEOPLE HEAR that I'm a sex therapist and Xander and I run a sex therapy business together, they immediately assume we have a wildly kinky sex life. But here's what physical intimacy can look like between us if we're not careful:

One of us asks, "Hey, do you want to have sex?"

The other person responds, "I guess. Can it be a quickie?"

We walk upstairs together and get the dogs situated in their bed before closing our bedroom door on them. We take our clothes off while standing up, then get onto Xander's side of the bed. Xander lies on his right side, I lie on my left. We kiss for a minute or two, then touch each other's genitals for another minute. We both want to be on the bottom, for reasons of sheer laziness, so we briefly tussle over who has to do the work of being on top. Usually it falls to the person who initiated. We have intercourse for a few minutes, and both of us focus on getting ourselves off. Once we're done, we clean ourselves up, then head back downstairs.

Not exactly thrilling, right? (Side note: I read this to Xander during the editing phase, and he responded, "I feel attacked.")

I asked our Instagram audience to share their stories of sex feeling routine and stale. I got thousands of responses. As I sifted through them, I couldn't help but laugh at how identical the stories were:

"We try to get it over with as quickly as possible."

"We have the same couple of positions we default to over and over again."

"There's approximately two minutes of foreplay."

"We default to the same 'what we know gets the job done' routine every time."

"We just do enough foreplay for me to get wet enough for penetration."

"It's the exact same thing. Every. Single. Time. I can't remember the last time we tried something new."

"It happens in this way because it's comfortable and not bad, and no one needs to really think about it."

Even the tone of all these descriptions is the same, despite being written by different people. You can *feel* the monotony.

It's frustratingly easy to fall into a sexual rut. With busy schedules, demanding jobs, kids, families, and never-ending responsibilities, your partner can slip to the bottom of your to-do list. (I'm powerless against these puns!) As much as you love your partner, and as much as you may be attracted to them, you're still going to find yourself mindlessly going through the motions in the bedroom.

This kind of sex feels safe. It's okay. It's not terrible. It's a "the devil you know is better than the devil you don't" type of situation. Remember my friend Emmy? She told me, "We keep doing the same routine because it feels too awkward to do something different. I'd rather do stuff I know 'works' than try something new and have it not be a good experience. Especially since our time together is so limited. Why risk it?"

"Risk" is the perfect word. What if you try something new and it goes terribly? What if you get embarrassed? What if it hurts? What if you suggest an idea and get judged by your partner? What if you discover that your sweet, mild-mannered husband secretly wants you to put diapers on him and pretend to nurse him? What if you discover that you actually like that, too?

But this kind of sex is slowly sapping the energy out of you and your relationship. It's the equivalent of eating white toast for breakfast every morning. It's fine. Sometimes it's surprisingly comforting or even tasty. But it's the same effing bread every single day. It's why I call the connection between enjoyment and desire from Conversation 3 the White Toast Problem. You're never going to wake up in the morning thinking, "I just can't *wait* to eat another piece of that white toast!"

There's also what I call the Inhibition Effect at play. Have you ever noticed that the longer you date someone, the more vanilla your sex life gets? Xander put his finger in my butt after only days of knowing me. But by the time we were a few years into dating, anal play had gone the way of the dinosaurs. For a lot of people, there's an inverse relationship between intimacy and adventurousness. It's as if as every year that passes, another item disappears from your sexual menu. It's a funny kind of twist on our old friend the Stranger; ironically, we feel more comfortable being uninhibited and wild when our partner feels more unknown to us.

Sexual routines are so easy to slip into that every couple should work to actively avoid this trap. But if bedroom boredom is your primary complaint with your sex life, this Sex Talk should be your starting place.

So how, exactly, do we talk about this in our relationships? How do we tell each other that we're weary of the same old routine, but at the same time we're too intimidated to shake it up? And how do we have any sort of conversation without hurting our partner's feelings, or putting pressure on ourselves to deliver nonstop novelty and excitement?

The Wrong Question

You already know the best antidote for sexual boredom: trying new things. It's no secret that when you shake up your routine—inside and outside of the bedroom—you get to see each other in a new light. It feels like you're dating each other again, still getting to know each other. Things feel fresh and new, instead of stale and predictable.

But if you're like most people, the way you broach the conversation about trying new things in the bedroom is by asking, "What's your fantasy?"

I remember asking Xander this very question early in our relationship. It took a lot of courage to ask, but I was excited for his answer. I was ready for his long wish list of sexual adventures, so we could start working our way through them and checking them off, one by one.

Much to my horror, he responded, "Uh . . . I don't really have any."

My heart stopped.

He continued. "Do *you* have any? I'm open to do whatever you want to do."

"Oh, not really. I'm happy with what we're doing!" I blurted out.

The conversation came to a complete standstill, but my mind started racing. Did Xander really not have *any* fantasies? He was fine just continuing to do the exact same thing, over and over again? I had been relying on him for some inspiration! Did I even have any fantasies myself? There were a few things I had thought about trying, but if Xander was happy with what we were doing, maybe I shouldn't mention them. After all, I wouldn't want him judging me or thinking I was weird for being interested in . . .

Things might have continued down a pretty monotonous path had I not had a moment of inspiration a few weeks later. I reminded myself, *This is the guy who put his finger in my butt. He has got to be into other stuff.* I started thinking about the word "fantasy"; maybe it was the wrong word to be using. After all, I wouldn't even describe my own curiosities as full-blown fantasies. So, a few days later, I asked Xander, "What's one thing you're curious about trying in the bedroom with me?" *Bingo*! I got a response!

Years later, after talking about the word "fantasy" with thousands of people, I can confidently say that we're focusing on the wrong question. I asked our Instagram audience, "Do you have any fantasies?" and 70 percent said no. Many of us think that "fantasy" means "an incredibly elaborate and detailed scene involving role-playing and story arcs that I think about *constantly* and makes me orgasm just to think about." For example, "Okay, so we're in eighteenth-century England. I'm a duchess, and you're my husband's sexy, younger butler. He goes on a business trip to collect the tax payments from the townspeople. A huge storm rolls in, and I'm frightened by the lightning and thunder. . . ." If you know you're completely into eighteenth-century thunderstorms (or the aforementioned diapers), that's awesome! I love that for you! But if the word "fantasy" doesn't resonate with you, that doesn't mean you have no interests or curiosities whatsoever.

The other funny thing about "What's your fantasy?" is that it's often a lazy question! It reminds me again of the dreaded "What do you want for dinner?" debacle. You think you're being polite and letting your partner choose what they want to eat, but it actually feels like a burden to your partner to have to come up with an answer they think you'll both love. That was certainly the case for me. I felt embarrassed sharing the things I was curious about trying with Xander, so I wanted to punt the responsibility to him.

Instead, I encourage you to use the same question I asked Xander: "What's one thing you're *curious* about trying?" And come prepared with an answer of your own.

It's much more fun to approach sexual interests from a place of curiosity than of certainty, as in, "I guarantee you this is something that wildly turns me on, and I've kept it a secret all these years."

And remember what we talked about in the last chapter—that you can ask for something without being positive that you'll like it? "What's your fantasy?" implies that you already know you'll love it, whereas "What are you curious about?" leaves the space for your reaction to be, "Hmm, yeah, I'm glad we tried that, but I don't think I'd do that again."

The Yes, No, Maybe Test

If the idea of coming up with something you're curious about trying *still* feels intimidating to you, I've got your back! It can be helpful to start with specific sex acts to evaluate, rather than feeling pressure to come up with completely new, exciting ideas from scratch. On the following pages, you'll find a long (but not complete!) list of activities that you could do in the bedroom.

You'll also see that there are three categories: Yesses, Maybes, and Nos.

This exercise is similar to the Red Lights, Yellow Lights, Green Lights boundary exercise from Chapter 3. Your Yesses are things you already know you enjoy. Your Nos are things you know you would never do. The Maybes are where it gets interesting. You might consider them based on the circumstances. You might be interested in trying one certain aspect of the activity, but not the whole thing. Maybe you would try it if you had a partner who was really into it, or if you could set it up in a certain way. Or maybe you're not interested in trying it now, but you might be open to it in the future. I like including this category because it gives you the opportunity to reexamine your boundaries.

My friend Francesca and I talked about her Maybes multiple times. When I introduce the concept to her, she thinks it's hysterical, telling me, "Okay, so like piss play . . . Urine plus sex does not sound appealing to me in the slightest. But if Jake was really turned on by it . . . I *might* consider it. Could we do it in the shower, for easy clean-up? Could I just pee a little on his foot or his leg?" A few weeks later, Francesca has an example that feels more serious. "Jake wants me to send him nudes. That wasn't really a thing when we started dating. It sounds kinda hot, but I'm also nervous about the photos leaking or someone accidentally seeing them."

For each item on the list, go through and decide if that activity is a Yes, No, or Maybe for you at this point in time.

You and your partner should each fill out a copy of the worksheet individually. Then come together to discuss your answers to each item. You can go through the list all at once or one page at a time. Your only rule for this process is that neither of you are allowed to say anything negative about the other person's interests—especially if your partner is into something that you're not, or vice versa. No jokes, no shaming, no shocked responses. Try your best to stay neutral. If you're nervous about how this part of the process will go, you can come up with an agreed-upon response beforehand, like "I respect that you're interested in that even though I'm not open to it."

Let's Do This

Here's your game plan for different combinations of responses:

- If you're both Yes, awesome! Add it to your to-do list.
- If you're both No, great, you don't ever have to do that thing.
- If one person is Yes or Maybe and one person is No, that item goes on your joint No list. There may be some sadness or disappointment from the partner who was the Yes or Maybe, but it's important to respect your partner's boundaries. (And remember, no shaming.)
- If you're both Maybe or one Yes and one Maybe, this is where it gets really interesting. Here are some questions to help you guys figure out what to do with that item:

"Is there an aspect of this that we're curious about, even if we're not interested in doing the whole thing?"
"What makes us feel nervous or uncertain about this?"
"What circumstances would make us feel more comfortable?"
"How could we adjust this to make it more comfortable?"
"Should we table this for now and come back to it in the future?"

The Yes, No, Maybe Test

Cuddling	YES	NO	MAYBE
Massaging my partner	YES	NO	MAYBE
Getting a massage	YES	NO	MAYBE
Kissing	YES	NO	MAYBE
Kissing with tongue	YES	NO	MAYBE
Kissing all over my partner's body	YES	NO	MAYBE
Having my body kissed	YES	NO	MAYBE
PDA	YES	NO	MAYBE
Talking about desires with my partner	YES	NO	MAYBE
Sending suggestive emails or text messages to my partner	YES	NO	MAYBE
Receiving suggestive emails or text messages from my partner	YES	NO	MAYBE
Sending sexy pictures to my partner	YES	NO	MAYBE
Receiving sexy pictures from my partner	YES	NO	MAYBE
Having phone sex (audio only)	YES	NO	MAYBE
Having a sexy video chat	YES	NO	MAYBE
Playing with my partner's breasts	YES	NO	MAYBE
Having my partner play with my breasts	YES	NO	MAYBE
Playing with my partner's nipples	YES	NO	MAYBE
Having my partner play with my nipples	YES	NO	MAYBE
Playing with my partner's balls	YES	NO	MAYBE
My partner playing with my balls	YES	NO	MAYBE
Listening to my partner moan	YES	NO	MAYBE
Moaning	YES	NO	MAYBE
Talking dirty	YES	NO	MAYBE
Playing music during sex	YES	NO	MAYBE
Dry humping	YES	NO	MAYBE
Outercourse (dry humping without clothes)	YES	NO	MAYBE

Giving hand jobs	YES	NO	MAYBE
Receiving hand jobs	YES	NO	MAYBE
Masturbating solo	YES	NO	MAYBE
Watching my partner masturbate	YES	NO	MAYBE
Masturbating in front of my partner	YES	NO	MAYBE
Masturbating together	YES	NO	MAYBE
Using lube on my partner	YES	NO	MAYBE
Having my partner use lube on me	YES	NO	MAYBE
Giving oral sex	YES	NO	MAYBE
Receiving oral sex	YES	NO	MAYBE
Having intercourse	YES	NO	MAYBE
Seeing my partner completely naked	YES	NO	MAYBE
Being completely naked in front of my partner	YES	NO	MAYBE
Being intimate outside of the bedroom	YES	NO	MAYBE
Being intimate in the shower and/or bathtub	YES	NO	MAYBE
Sex with the lights on	YES	NO	MAYBE
Sex in the dark	YES	NO	MAYBE
Morning sex	YES	NO	MAYBE
Afternoon sex	YES	NO	MAYBE
Evening sex	YES	NO	MAYBE
Having sex in a semipublic place	YES	NO	MAYBE
Reading erotic fiction on my own	YES	NO	MAYBE
Reading erotic fiction with my partner	YES	NO	MAYBE
Listening to audio erotica on my own	YES	NO	MAYBE
Listening to audio erotica with my partner	YES	NO	MAYBE
Watching porn solo	YES	NO	MAYBE
Watching porn together	YES	NO	MAYBE
Role-playing	YES	NO	MAYBE
Wearing costumes	YES	NO	MAYBE
Dominating my partner	YES	NO	MAYBE

Being dominated	YES	NO	MAYBE
Seeing my partner in lingerie	YES	NO	MAYBE
Wearing lingerie	YES	NO	MAYBE
Having an orgasm	YES	NO	MAYBE
Having multiple orgasms	YES	NO	MAYBE
Edging	YES	NO	MAYBE
(If your partner has a penis) Having my partner ejaculate somewhere they normally don't	YES	NO	MAYBE
(If you have a penis) Ejaculating somewhere I normally don't	YES	NO	MAYBE
Giving anal stimulation with my hands	YES	NO	MAYBE
Receiving anal stimulation from my partner's hands	YES	NO	MAYBE
Giving anal stimulation with my mouth	YES	NO	MAYBE
Receiving anal stimulation from my partner's mouth	YES	NO	MAYBE
Anal intercourse	YES	NO	MAYBE
Playing with a sex toy alone	YES	NO	MAYBE
Watching my partner use a sex toy	YES	NO	MAYBE
Having my partner watch me use a sex toy	YES	NO	MAYBE
Playing with a sex toy together with my partner	YES	NO	MAYBE
Having period sex	YES	NO	MAYBE
Having a quickie	YES	NO	MAYBE
Trying new sex positions	YES	NO	MAYBE
Having a threesome	YES	NO	MAYBE
Having group sex	YES	NO	MAYBE
Photographing or videotaping us having sex	YES	NO	MAYBE
Spanking my partner	YES	NO	MAYBE
Being spanked by my partner	YES	NO	MAYBE
Scratching my partner	YES	NO	MAYBE
Having my partner scratch me	YES	NO	MAYBE
Pulling my partner's hair	YES	NO	MAYBE
Having my hair pulled by my partner	YES	NO	MAYBE

Biting my partner	YES	NO	MAYBE
Having my partner bite me	YES	NO	MAYBE
Choking my partner	YES	NO	MAYBE
Being choked by my partner	YES	NO	MAYBE
Slapping my partner in the face	YES	NO	MAYBE
Being slapped in the face by my partner	YES	NO	MAYBE
Pain play	YES	NO	MAYBE
Restraining my partner	YES	NO	MAYBE
Being restrained by my partner	YES	NO	MAYBE
Blindfolding my partner	YES	NO	MAYBE
Being blindfolded by my partner	YES	NO	MAYBE
Performing double penetration on my partner	YES	NO	MAYBE
Experiencing double penetration from my partner	YES	NO	MAYBE
Calling my partner names (whore, slut, bad girl/boy, sissy, etc.)	YES	NO	MAYBE
Being called names by my partner	YES	NO	MAYBE

Obviously, some of the items on this list are more intense than others, so I want to remind you that your likes and wants in the bedroom don't need to be elaborate at all. They can be as small as enjoying deep kisses or back tickles. You don't get a higher grade for being willing to try pain play or participate in an orgy.

"How do we actually try new things?"

So many people hear the suggestion to mix things up in the bedroom and think they need to immediately draft a Dominant/submissive contract, like they saw in *Fifty Shades of Grey*. But you do not need to jump immediately into the deep end of the kinky pool! The best way to try new things in the bedroom is to make *small* changes. That will increase your confidence and motivation to keep exploring.

First, decide how frequently you'd like to try something new. My suggestion is to pick a schedule that feels totally manageable at first. Certainly not every time you have sex.

Next, take your to-do list and order it in terms of least intimidating to most intimidating. Pick the least-intimidating thing and make a specific game plan for when you're going to do it.

From there, you can try a few options:

- Work through your list in order. This works well if you like knowing what to expect.
- If you want some surprise, print out the ideas you currently feel comfortable doing on slips of paper, fold them up, and put them in a jar on your bedside table. Pick one at random to try out in the moment.
- Or pick your activity earlier in the day, so as to build anticipation for later that night.

If you want to surprise each other with something new, you can go through your to-do list and decide which items you'd be fine with your partner springing on you in the moment, and which ones you'd want to agree beforehand to explore. For example, maybe you'd feel fine with your partner surprising you with some light spanking, but you'd want a heads-up before anal play.

For trying more complex ideas, break the activity down into baby steps.

Let's say you and your partner are both interested in going to a sex club, but you're feeling pretty nervous about it. Instead of pressuring yourselves to have a wild night that very next weekend, here are some ways you could ease into it:

- Research the sex clubs in your area.
- Listen to a podcast about sex clubs.
- Watch erotica or porn about sex clubs.
- Look for online forums of people talking about their sex-club experiences.
- Talk dirty about what you would see and experience at a sex club, while it's just the two of you.
- Go to a sex club, but just watch the first time.

Not only is it so much less intimidating to approach fantasies in this way, but it's also useful and sexy! A lot of people start taking baby steps toward a fantasy, only to realize that they're not actually that into it. Or doing all the baby steps can increase the anticipation and excitement, making the actual fantasy even more fun when it does eventually happen.

Navigating Sexual Perfectionism

Let's return to our conversation about Sexual Perfectionism from Part One. Remember how I said that perfectionism is one of the biggest impediments to trying something new in the bedroom? Let's meet Zoya and Akio. They both come from sexually conservative cultures, but they don't want the sexless marriages they each saw their parents endure. Zoya and Akio had a lot of natural chemistry in their early years together, but their frequency dropped off a cliff after having kids, and it finally scared them enough to seek sex therapy. As is the case with almost all my clients, the frequency isn't the real problem; the quality of the sex they're having is. (Have you noticed that there's no Sex Talk about frequency?) I learn that Zoya and Akio have intercourse in Missionary position every time because it's the only position she's ever been able to have an orgasm in. They've tried a couple other positions, but Zoya didn't get anywhere close.

"We go in so optimistic that we'll find a new position, and it's devastating when it doesn't immediately work," she tells me. "At this point it's easier to default to what works rather than deal with the disappointment and tears that come with trying something new. It takes all the fun out of exploring when I end up in tears afterward."

Zoya is so wrapped up in the idea that she should *immediately* be able to orgasm in a brand-new position that she gets "devastated," cries, and shuts down if it doesn't happen. They're having Missionary sex—even though they're both bored by the monotony of using one position—because they're too afraid of new things not being perfect right away.

But here's the thing: Whenever you try something new, it's almost certainly *not* going to go exactly how you want it to.

"The very first time the two of you tried Missionary, did it go perfectly?" I ask them. They both stare at me. "I'm willing to bet that it took time for you to make that position so successful."

I tell them about my First Pancake rule. You know how when you make pancakes, the first one always turns out kind of strange? You might still eat it, but compared to the last pancake you make, the first one is always a weirdo. It's the same with sex. Before trying anything new in the bedroom—and certainly before acting on any elaborate desires—it's a good idea to lower the stakes. Say something like, "I'm glad we both want to try this out. I want to be clear that it's fine if it doesn't end up being as fun as we want it to be. Let's try to take the pressure off of making it *perfect*, especially the first time." You can even make a little joke out of seeing how weird your First Pancake will be. You can give a name to the sex sessions in which you decide to do something new, like Sexploration or Sexperimentation, to further take the pressure off.

I also encourage you to use my Third Time's the Charm guideline for sexual exploration: Give yourself three times to try something new before deciding whether or not you like it. Of course, if the new activity causes you any sort of emotional or physical pain, or you're certain you don't ever want to try it again, you don't have to repeat it.

Let's Do This

After you try something new, wait until at least the next day to check in about it.

First, tell each other, "I'm really proud of us for trying something new. I know not all of our experiments will be home runs, but I appreciate us both for being vulnerable and stretching outside of our comfort zones."

Next, ask each other:

"What did you enjoy about the new thing?"
"Would you want to try this again?"

If you didn't like your experiment, a simple "Nope!" is enough. Unless it brought up a safety issue or helped you learn something important about yourself, there's no need to dissect what you didn't love.

Sharing Your Desires

So far, I've been offering advice for switching things up in the bedroom if you don't have any curiosities or fantasies in mind. But if there's something specific that you want to try with your partner, one of my favorite tricks is the Dream Scheme. Tell your partner, "I had such an interesting dream last night about [fill in the blank]. It was surprisingly sexy. . . ." This gives you the perfect opportunity to gauge your partner's initial reaction to your idea. It *is* a small lie, which I normally wouldn't recommend, but it's in the service of having a healthier sex life, and it can help you build up the confidence to make more direct requests in the future. And if we want to get technical, a fantasy and a daydream aren't too different. If your partner responds neutrally or positively, you can continue with something like, "I had never really thought about doing that before, but after that dream, I have to admit that I'm kind of curious."

Let's Do This

Here are some other conversation starters for making requests in the bedroom:

"There's this thing I've always wanted to try, but I've been waiting until I found the right person."

"I'm not sure I'd actually like this, but I've always been a little curious about trying . . ."

"What did you fantasize about when you were a teenager? I fantasized about . . ."

"I feel really vulnerable sharing this with you, but I'm doing it because I trust you so much. You know what sounds kind of sexy to me?"

"Have you ever thought about doing . . ."

"I saw this movie that had a scene where the actors were doing . . . Would you ever do something like that?"

People often worry about being judged for their desires, regardless of how kinky or tame those desires actually are. I've had clients feel nervous about asking to spend more time kissing or requesting a massage. People have told me they feel anxious about asking for the very same things their partner has already asked them for! So, here's the most important thing that I want you to understand: as long as everyone enthusiastically consents, and you're not trying to manipulate or hurt anyone, your desires, wants, likes, and fantasies are perfectly normal, valid, and acceptable. Period.

You want your partner to tie you up? That's fine! You want your partner to call you a dirty little slut? That's fine! You want your partner to have sex with another man while you watch? That's fine!

And let me take that one step further: you *deserve* to ask for your desires, wants, likes, and fantasies. You deserve to have sex that is *for you*!

Your partner is going to have their own set of boundaries, and your partner very well may be a hard no on some of your requests. You're never going to find a partner whose sexual interests completely overlap with yours. But another person's boundaries don't take away from the fact that your desires are valid and worthy and deserving of your asking for them. In other words, even if your partner says "Absolutely not," that doesn't mean you shouldn't have asked or that your desire was wrong or bad.

If you're worried about your partner's judging you for your curiosities and desires, your first step is to stop judging *yourself*. We tell ourselves we can't ask for a certain thing in the bedroom or give a piece of feedback because our partner will react poorly. But the reality is that we're projecting our fears onto our partner and are avoiding confronting it within ourselves.

This might sound silly at first, but I encourage you to think about your likes and desires the same way you think about your food preferences. (Yes, another food metaphor!) It doesn't "mean" anything about you as a person if you love mushrooms or if you don't like blue cheese, just like it doesn't "mean" anything if you love giving oral sex or if you don't love Cowgirl position. And our preferences can change from day to day. One day you might be in the mood for slow, sensual sex, just like you might be in the mood for a juicy, bacon-topped cheeseburger. And then the next day, slow, sensual sex could sound like the last thing you would possibly want, just like a cheeseburger could sound heavy and unappetizing.

You wouldn't feel embarrassed to ask your partner if they were interested in having Thai food tonight, would you? Even if your partner said, "I dunno. Thai food doesn't sound great to me right now," you'd still feel fine about the fact that it had sounded good to you. You might have a partner who's a vegetarian, and it might be a bummer that they don't want to try caviar with you. But that doesn't mean there was anything wrong with your wanting to try caviar.

I'll give you a sex-related example. I have a fantasy about being forced to have sex, commonly called a rape fantasy. This is actually one of the top female fantasies, so I know I'm not alone. (Before I get into my personal story, I want to make it clear that almost no one fantasizes about *actually* being raped, since that's an incredibly traumatic and violating experience. Instead, I prefer to call this a *ravishment* fantasy. It's about someone taking control and bossing you around, but in a safe and fully consensual way.) Like most women, I've felt pretty embarrassed about this fantasy, so it took me a few years to bring it up with Xander, and I needed the Dream Scheme to do it.

Xander's initial response wasn't a great one. He didn't overtly shame me, but he said something along the lines of, "I just don't think I could ever do that. Even though I would know I'm pretending, it doesn't make me feel good to think about raping you." I felt that initial wave of shame and embarrassment at first, and I wished I hadn't said anything. But I tried to remind myself that Xander has his own random set of desires and boundaries, and just because they're different from my random set, that didn't make mine wrong.

I eventually shared with Xander that I felt embarrassed about mentioning it, and he reassured me that he wasn't judging me for having the curiosity. He said he was actually judging *himself* for not being into it! It turned into a real bonding experience for us both.

So, look, your partner *wants* to pleasure you. They want to know what you desire and like. They may even be *desperate* to know! I'm sure that you can think of plenty of times when your partner has asked for your feedback or has asked you to tell them what you want. Try to remember those times when you're feeling worried about sharing. You can even talk to your partner about the fact that you feel nervous, and you can say something like, "I know you've asked me to tell you what I want and like in the past. It has been hard for me, but I really want to try. I'm in the middle of figuring it all out, but are you still open to my being more vocal?"

The Other Half with Xander:
"But what if my partner does get insecure?"

Let me set the scene—it was a Sunday in the early years of our relationship, and we were lazily sitting on the couch watching football. As Vanessa was staring wistfully at the screen, she asked me, "What if you role-played a football player with me?" I immediately felt a wave of fear and anxiety wash over me because I looked *nothing* like the average football player at the time. I was imagining myself going out to buy some oversized shoulder pads and a jersey, which—in my head—would look absolutely ridiculous on my non-athletic physique. For most of my life I had been quite long and lanky, struggling to put on much-needed pounds regardless of how much I ate. But suddenly I was acutely aware of the impact that extreme lack of exercise and sixty-hour workweeks (hello, stress eating!) were having on my twenty-four-year-old body. I was getting pudgy, and I didn't feel good about it.

I quickly shut down her request, telling her it sounded like too much work. I desperately wanted to just forget about the entire interaction, but I found I couldn't stop myself from wondering if there was something else behind it. Was I not sexy enough for her? Did she wish I was in better shape? That I was more confident and assertive?

I tell you that story to be honest with you: sharing your fantasies *does* have the possibility of bringing up some insecurities for your partner. While you'll never be able to be in complete control of how your partner reacts to something you share, you can do your part to set your partner up for success. A simple way to do this is to share the reasons why you want to try this certain thing *with your partner*, specifically. Maybe you think they'd look sexy in a football uniform. Maybe they're the only person who has helped you feel safe enough to explore your fantasies. Whatever it is, share with your partner why they are a crucial part of your sexual desires instead of just playing a role that any other person could play. You want to make your requests and curiosities feel personal to your partner.

Looping back to the football-player example, I would have been much more open to Vanessa's idea if she had said something along the lines of:

- "I have a fantasy that I'm a little embarrassed about—in fact, you're the first person I've felt comfortable sharing this with."
- "I'm not usually attracted to football players, but I'm so attracted to you that I was thinking it could be sexy to pretend you were a football player pushing me around in bed—would you be open to role-playing that sometime?"
- And if I had responded with any anxiety or worry: "For me, it has nothing to do with actually looking the part, and we don't need to get any props. I think it would just be fun to pretend together and enjoy it!"

Had Vanessa shared this fantasy using some of my suggestions, I might even have been excited about it! It would have felt really good to know she was a bit embarrassed, too, but was still comfortable sharing it with me. And knowing that *I* was the person she wanted, rather than someone who looked like Fred Warner on the 49ers, would have helped build up my confidence in taking on that role.

"What if my partner is turned on by something that doesn't turn me on?"

I asked our Instagram audience: "Do you and your partner have different sexual interests and curiosities?" A whopping 90 percent of respondents said yes! With numbers like those, it's inevitable that you'll have a sexual interest that your partner doesn't share, or vice versa.

So, what do you do if your partner tells you they want to try something, but you're not into it? Here are my suggestions:

- Treat your partner and their fantasy with respect. Say something like, "I know it takes a lot of courage and trust to be honest about your desires, and I appreciate you being so vulnerable with me."
- Get a better sense of how important this particular activity is. Ask questions like "Is this something that you want to try in real life, or did you just want to share the idea with me?" or "How central is this fantasy to your sexual expression and fulfillment?" and, "What level of involvement were you hoping for from me?" For example, there can be a huge difference between feeling bummed out that you'll never get to suck on your partner's toes, versus never being able to explore your bi-curiosity.
- See if there's a part of the fantasy that does interest you. Remember my advice to break fantasies down into baby steps? Maybe you're not open to filming yourselves have sex, but you would be okay taking some tasteful boudoir photos.

What Happens When It Doesn't Work Out?

Getting back to that little ravishment fantasy I mentioned earlier, Xander and I felt really good about the way we handled that conversation, and he ended up coming around to the idea of trying it out in real life.

Unfortunately, I hadn't yet figured out my own baby-step advice, so we jumped right in. (The vast majority of my advice to you in this book comes from having done the exact opposite in my own sex life! I am my own guinea pig.)

It . . . didn't go great. It was awkward and uncomfortable for both of us, and Xander asked to stop after a few minutes. This is the reality of sexual fantasies. They can be super sexy in our heads, but in real life they don't always work out exactly how we imagined them.

It was a bit embarrassing in the moment for both of us. But it also helped us learn some important details and nuance about this fantasy:

- There were certain acts that Xander realized he didn't want to do, like choking me. That wasn't a central part of the fantasy for me, so I was fine with it.
- I had gone quiet during sex, but that made Xander feel nervous. He wanted to know that I actually was enjoying myself, even though we were role-playing.
- I realized that I didn't need to have an elaborate setup. Some people like having full story arcs to a ravishment fantasy, like having their partner "break in" to their house wearing a ski mask. I realized I just liked Xander to be bossy and dominant in the moment.

Just because your First Pancake is weird, that doesn't mean you should give up on it altogether! Xander and I decided to leave the full ravishment fantasy in my own fantasies, but we have brought elements of it into our regular sex life, and we're both pretty happy about that outcome.

"My partner and I talked about trying new things in the bedroom, and neither of us wants to. Is that okay?"

If both you and your partner are perfectly content with your sex life as is, you absolutely don't need to force yourselves to experiment. My suggestion is to ask each other this question (if you haven't already): *"Why* don't we want to try anything new?" If you dig deep and allow yourself to be honest, you may discover that the answer might be informed by internalized negative messages about sex, Sexual Perfectionism, or even trauma. For example, "Exploring new things in the bedroom has never felt safe to me." Or you may discover that the answer is pretty simple and straightforward: "It's just not my jam." If that's the case, then great!

Just make sure to revisit this conversation every few years or so, and make sure you're both still on board. You want to make space for the reality that things may change.

"My husband and I both agreed to experiment with anal sex. He loved it, and I hated it. I'm trying not to be judgmental, but I hated it so much that it does make me judge him a little bit for liking it. What do I say when he asks me to do it again?"

It's okay for you and your partner to have completely different experiences with the same sexual act. And it's understandable that your reaction to it is so strong that it's allowing some judgment to come creeping in. The key is to not share that with your partner, because sharing it could set up a dynamic whereby it doesn't feel safe to suggest or try new things.

Take the initiative and bring up the topic of anal sex before he asks for it again. Say something like, "I'm really glad you and I are exploring in the bedroom together. It feels fun and exciting, and I want to keep doing it! I've been thinking about our experience doing anal, and it just wasn't my thing.

I know you liked it, so I'm bummed that I don't feel the same. But I'd love to pick something else for us to explore together."

This experience also drives home the importance of having a Post-Game discussion after trying something new. If you create a container where you can safely and proactively say how it felt for you, you won't get into a situation like this, where you're dreading what will happen the next time your partner asks you to do it.

"Vulva owner here. I suggested bringing a toy into the bedroom, and he said, 'Eew, no, we shouldn't need something like that.' I feel hurt and shut down. What now?"

First of all, kudos to you for getting up the courage to make that suggestion. I'm sorry your partner had a negative reaction to it. I know it feels easier to stay shut down, but this is definitely a conversation the two of you need to have again.

Sexual shame can sometimes cause us to react a lot more negatively to suggestions than we actually feel. When you're both in a good mood, loop back around and say something like this: "Hey, I want to talk about the vibrator conversation again. I want you and I to have a relationship where we can explore sex without shame. I'm sure you didn't mean to hurt my feelings, but I felt ashamed when you said 'eew' about using a vibrator. We're different people and we're allowed to have different boundaries, but I don't want either of us to ever make each other feel bad if our boundaries aren't in alignment. I'd like to talk about vibrators again, but without any shaming. Can we do that?"

If you and your partner haven't already had discussions about how vulva orgasm really works, make sure to read Conversation 4 (chapter 8) together. A vibrator can be an excellent way to ensure that your pleasure is given as much priority as your partner's.

My hope is that your partner's reaction was more about his insecurity than about his judgment. Sometimes men worry that their female partner wanting to use a vibrator means they're not "good in bed." You can assure him that your desire to play with a vibrator says nothing about his sexual skill, and then focus on why it's fun for you to explore new activities *with* him.

JUST THE TIP(S):

- It's natural to fall into a routine in your sex life, even if you're painfully bored by said routine, but trying new things in the bedroom is the best way to keep your sex life spicy for years to come.
- "What's your fantasy?" is the wrong question to ask.
- The Yes, No, Maybe test will help you identify the specific new things you and your partner want to try in the bedroom together.
- Take baby steps when trying anything new, and remember the First Pancake rule. Don't expect it to go perfectly the first time (or the first few times).
- It's normal for you and your partner to have your own curiosities, so don't judge yourselves or each other for any differences.

Congratulations—you've now completed your five Sex Talks! I hope you've developed a richer understanding of your sexual self and have enjoyed the journey of deepening intimacy with your partner. I'm incredibly proud of you, and I'm excited for how your sex life will continue to unfold!

I know that, just like sex, conversation doesn't always go the way we want it to. So, in the next chapter, I'll give you tips for getting back on track if things went haywire at any point.

Part Three

KEEPING THE
TWIN FLAMES
ALIVE FOR LIFE

CHAPTER 10

WHAT TO DO WHEN CONVERSATIONS GO OFF THE RAILS

DESPITE YOUR BEST intentions and preparations, you're still going to have moments when you seem to black out and lose all the communication skills you've ever learned. Xander and I had a miscommunication not thirty minutes ago, when he made a suggestion for how to make this book better, and I took it as his telling me it's not good enough. Sex and relationships are just hard to talk about! There's a reason why I wrote this book, and why you picked it up. So, let's talk about how to get back on track if "The Talk" turns into "The Fight."

What Is Conflict, Anyway?

Most of us go to great lengths to avoid getting into any sort of disagreement with our partner—or anyone else in our life, for that matter. And when we do have a fight, the negative feelings can linger for days. But I want to reframe what conflict actually is, because there's just no way to avoid it. All couples have arguments. Us included.

I like to think of conflicts as missed attempts at intimacy. The two of you have the desire to be close and connected, but your intentions go awry in some unfortunate way. Having an argument doesn't mean you're a terrible fit for each other or that your relationship is doomed. Instead, it's an *opportunity* to clear up misunderstandings and to understand yourselves and each other more deeply. If handled properly, disagreements can actually bring you closer together because you build trust when you can handle each other's stuff.

In the middle of writing this book, Xander and I also moved. (Pro tip: I do *not* recommend this!) It was a stressful time for us, made even more stressful by the fact that the professional movers we had hired to transport us from Los Angeles to Santa Barbara didn't show up on the day of our move and weren't responding to calls or texts. After ninety minutes had passed, Xander came out into the backyard, where I was trying to calm myself down with some deep breaths.

"Hey, Babe," he said. I instantly knew something was up. "So, uh, I double-checked the contract I signed, and, uh, it looks like I accidentally scheduled the move for tomorrow, not for today."

Time stood still as I tried to process this information. *He booked the move for the wrong day.* How could he have made such a boneheaded mistake? How could he mix up the dates? How could he not have double-checked the contract before signing it, much less before today? I didn't trust what was going to come out of my mouth, so I just stayed silent for ten painful minutes. I tend to clam up when I'm upset, and I know myself well enough to know that I could have kept up the silent treatment all day long while Xander begged for forgiveness.

But there was something about the sheer ridiculousness of having your entire life packed up and nowhere to move it to that eventually made me burst into laughter. I was able to look over at Xander and see him as a human who made a mistake, as simple as that. I knew in my heart that his intent was to make the move as smooth as possible, and he was able to acknowledge that his actions had a hugely negative impact on me (as well as him). And although my initial reaction to his nervous confession had been anger, I was able to see it as a bid for connection. He had made a mistake, he was in pain, and he didn't want to be alone. We gave each other a big hug, we acknowledged how stressful the last few weeks had been, and we made a Plan B for the move.

Now, let me walk you through some potential scenarios that may come up for you and your partner in your sexual communication journey, and give you my best advice for dealing with each of them.

If Your Partner Doesn't Engage

During any of your Sex Talks, your partner might nod along and say things like "Sure" or "That sounds fine," but not participate in a more meaningful way.

Let's first give your partner the benefit of the doubt and assume that they're feeling overwhelmed. In most relationships, there tends to be one partner who takes the lead in wanting to work on the partnership. (You might even say they carry the Mental Load of the relationship.)

Since you're the one who picked up this book, that's probably you, so your partner may just need some time to catch up. You can say something like, "I know this is a challenging topic to talk about. It sure is for me! I've had the opportunity to think about this more since I've been reading this book. How about I give you more time to process, because I'm genuinely interested in hearing what you have to say about [the specific topic at hand]. Then we can reconvene at [suggest a specific time]." You're making it okay for your partner to take time, and you're assuring them that you're genuinely interested in their perspective.

If your partner still seems disengaged, pick one specific baby step that you want to start with together. For example, "I'd love for us to read this chapter together this week. We don't have to do any of the exercises yet; let's just read it first." This is another way to help minimize any overwhelm that they may be feeling. Make a specific suggestion about the timing, too.

Okay, so maybe you read Vanessa's suggestions here and thought, "Yeah, those ideas are great and all, but the problem with my partner is that they just don't care." I want to tell you, from personal experience, that that's almost certainly *not* the case! There's probably a lot that's swirling through your partner's head, and what you're perceiving as apathy is actually their attempt to process and make sense of it all.

In the past, Vanessa has made requests of me, and I know I have come off as being disengaged. But in reality, here are some of the things that were going through my head at the time:

- I felt "behind" because she brought up something that sounded serious or important, but I hadn't noticed or thought about it yet.
- I got embarrassed about what it must say about me—for example, "I must be so boring because she wants more Doggystyle, but I'm happy sticking with Missionary."
- The thing she was asking for felt really challenging to me, so I thought, *I'm just going to run out the clock and hope she forgets about this.*
- I felt like a little kid being scolded, even if Vanessa wasn't literally scolding me or even telling me I had done something "wrong." Sometimes our subconscious can just get reminded of a hurtful time from childhood!
- I thought only one of us could be right or get what we want, so it would be better for me to dig in my heels or avoid her request.

In all these examples, I would have appeared to be anywhere from totally disengaged—at best—to a complete jerk. But in reality, I was just struggling with some big emotions that were coming up for me! So, the bottom line is to remember that your partner cares about you and your relationship.

They're just working with different timing, and they might need some more space to work through their emotions, too.

If Your Partner Stonewalls You

Stonewalling is a more extreme version of disengagement. It's when your partner completely withdraws, shuts down, or refuses to communicate. Stonewalling can be done without words (giving you the cold shoulder or an icy glare), or it can include phrases like, "I'm not talking about this." In my professional experience, men tend to stonewall far more often than women.

It really sucks to be on the receiving end of stonewalling. It also really sucks to be the one *doing* the stonewalling! I know it might seem like your partner is being an unfeeling robot, but as a psychotherapist, I can tell you that what's actually going on is that they're feeling scared and vulnerable. They're being flooded by emotion, and they're paralyzed. Your partner is putting their walls up as an ill-conceived protective mechanism.

You might be frustrated that your partner won't respond, but I want you to know that human beings are *incapable* of responding when we're that distressed. What's happening to your partner is called "emotional flooding," and it has a paralyzing effect on our bodies. We lose our capacity to access our thoughts and emotions. Our hearing literally shuts down. We can dissociate from our physical bodies. It's not that your partner *won't* respond, it's that they *can't*. And the harder you push for them to engage, the less capable they are of doing so.

The best way to address stonewalling is to talk about this dynamic when things are calm, and to make a game plan for what to do when either you or your partner experiences emotional flooding. We all get emotionally flooded from time to time, so you can approach it as a team instead of making your partner feel like something is horribly wrong with them. Show them this section of the chapter and tell them you now understand more about what's happening for them in moments like these.

When either of you experience emotional flooding, you need to step away from the conflict for at least twenty minutes. And you can't ruminate on the argument during that break. (In other words, it doesn't count as a time-out if all you're doing is thinking about the fight.) Instead, practice self-soothing by taking deep breaths, moving around, getting outside, feeling your feet on the ground, listening to music, or doing a mindless task. Only after taking this break will you be able to come back and have a productive conversation.

It helps to devise a specific plan for how you're going to take this time-out. Instead of saying, "I'm not talking about this," you or your partner could say, "I'm feeling overwhelmed. I'm going to take a few minutes to myself, then I'll come back to you and we can continue this conversation." Or, "I'm feeling overloaded. I don't want to do the stonewalling thing, so just give me a minute to gather myself." You can even come up with a code word or physical signal that means the same thing.

Of course, stonewalling can become a much bigger issue if your partner does it often or refuses to make a game plan when things are calm, so couples therapy may be a necessary step.

If Your Partner Gets Defensive

Let's take it up a notch and talk about what to do if your partner won't let you share your experience, or your partner tries to turn the tables and focus on your wrongdoings instead of their own words or actions. Defensiveness can sound like "But *you're* the one who always turns *me* down for sex" or "I've been trying to get you to talk about our sex life for years!"

The best way to stop defensiveness in its tracks is to validate it. Let your partner know that you do care about their experience. I'll give you a heads-up: this is *not* going to feel great for you in the moment. When your partner gets defensive, it's so easy to feel argumentative in return, and then fights can escalate quickly. You might feel the temptation to holler something like "Why would I ever say yes to sex if the only way you ever initiate is by groping at me like a child? You *really* think that turns me on?" Before you know it, you're in an all-out brawl.

Instead, let your partner know that you hear, understand, and respect their perspective, even if it's wildly different from yours. (Skip ahead to the "Aim for Understanding, Not Agreement" section for more details.) Try something like this: "I can imagine that it must be really hard to get turned down. It's difficult for me to talk about, but I do want to hear what that has been like for you. Would you be open to sharing more about that with me? And would you be open to listening to what I'd like to share with you?" Remind your partner that you want to be on the same team by saying something like, "I know we love each other deeply and we both want to have a sex life that feels satisfying. We have some things to work on together, but I know we both really want to get there. Can we be a team?"

If Your Partner Uses Emotion to Deflect

Another way your partner might derail the conversation is by self-flagellating. Some people will blame themselves entirely and say things like "I'm such a horrible person. Why would you want to be with me?"

It's hard to see your partner beat themselves up, so you might take pity on your partner and say something like "No, you're wonderful, I love you! Forget what I said; I didn't mean it" or "It's really not that big a deal!" It might seem like your partner is suffering and needs your compassion. But in reality, they're being manipulative (whether or not they're aware of it) and using emotion to deflect rather than take any real responsibility.

If you get this kind of response from your partner, hold your ground gently but firmly. Say something like, "I don't think you're a horrible person, and I feel sad that you're going to that place within yourself. I want to be clear that I'm making this request of you, without making a judgment of you." You can also remind your partner that there are things you want to improve personally, too, but you don't think that makes you a bad person, either.

This can be a tricky dynamic to deal with on your own, so I'll put in another plug for couples therapy, especially if it's something that's happening often.

If It Turns into a Full-Blown Fight

There's no way around it: it sucks to argue. But let me remind you that Xander and I teach sexual communication for a living, and we *still* get into conflicts about intimacy. And we've had bad ones, too—like "book an emergency couples therapy session" bad. We survived, and you can survive, also. Here are the specific steps to walk through if a fight erupts:

Take a Break

One of Xander's and my major communication challenges is that we get stuck talking in circles. No one is saying anything new, and we're certainly not making any progress toward a resolution, but we can't seem to shut our mouths. If it feels like the conversation isn't going anywhere, put yourselves on a time-out. It's a similar approach to dealing with stonewalling. Sometimes just stepping away for ten minutes is enough.

This tip works best if you talk about it beforehand. Make an agreement that it's okay for anyone to ask for a time-out whenever they need one.

Some people get triggered by the word "break" because it sounds too close to "breakup." If that's the case for you, come up with a code word or specific phrase that you use to put a pause on the conversation. Saying "Fuzzy caterpillars" can feel a lot better in the moment than yelling, "Screw you, asshole, I'm taking a break!"

In the moment, remind each other of the purpose of the break. You can say something like "I need to gather my thoughts so I can share them with you more effectively" or "I want to slow myself down so I can be a better communicator." Or even, "I want to take a time-out so I can make sure I don't say something I don't mean in the heat of the moment." This helps you both feel better about putting things on pause.

The most important thing to do is to tell each other that you're going to come back to the topic at hand. Taking a break doesn't mean you're ending the conversation right there; you *will* come back and finish the conversation. So, you may want to include that in your request by saying something like, "I need a ten-minute breather. Can we come back and finish the conversation after that?"

Feel Your Feelings

Most of us have no idea what to do with our emotions, so we get extremely uncomfortable when conflict inevitably stirs up the big ones. But here's the secret to feelings: the only way *out* is *through*. When we give ourselves permission to experience our emotions, they fade. When we fight our feelings, they get so much stronger. It's not our emotions themselves that are the problem; it's how we deal with them. (Remember how I walked Francesca through this when we were dealing with her Sexual Perfectionism?) So, give yourself permission to feel every single feeling that comes up for you, even the difficult ones.

Think about how this dynamic might have played out at other points in your life. Maybe there was a time when you were a little kid that you were scared about something, and your parents said, "Don't be such a baby." Did that make you feel less scared? No way! Or what about a time that you got into a fight with your partner and they said, "Don't be ridiculous." Did that make you feel more secure? Of course not!

All that your feelings really want is some validation. Permission to exist. That's strangely relatable, isn't it?

So, whenever you notice an emotion come up, take a second to identify and validate it. Researchers at UCLA's Social Cognitive Neuroscience

Laboratory found that the act of identifying our feelings makes them feel less intense.[1] I'll say to myself, "Okay, I'm feeling anxiety. I give my anxiety permission to be there."

Check Your Stories

We typically assign our own meanings to the things our partner says and does, and then we respond to those meanings that we've created. I'll give you an example: Let's say you asked your partner to make a reservation at a restaurant for date night, and they forgot to do it. Your brain is probably going to start thinking, *I guess my partner doesn't care about date night.* If you're feeling particularly sensitive, that thought can really snowball into things like, *My partner doesn't want to spend time with me. She must not love me anymore.* Cue a massive fight. But that's just the story you've created in your head; there could be a million other reasons why your partner forgot.

Instead, what you can do is share your story with your partner. Say something like, "When you forgot to make a reservation for date night, my mind started thinking that maybe it's because you don't care about our having quality time together. But I don't know if that's how you actually feel, so I wanted to ask."

You still get to share the feelings and insecurities that are coming to you, but you're doing it in a gentler way that allows your partner to respond. (By the way, this technique also works really well for preventing fights from occurring in the first place. If you can check your story before getting worked up about it, you can avoid a lot of heartache.)

No one likes being told how they feel. If your partner were to tell you, "You don't care about date night anymore," I'm sure you'd feel angry! Asking questions and allowing your partner to be the ultimate authority on their own feelings softens things up between the two of you.

And often there's a good explanation. Maybe your partner has been feeling stressed about taking care of their ailing parent. Maybe they thought they *had* made a reservation. Maybe they thought date night was the following week. Your stories and your meanings are frequently going to be wrong.

So, it's better to get them out there in a gentle way and correct your assumptions, rather than keeping them inside and feeling hurt and resentful.

Remind Yourselves That You're on the Same Team

Remember that it's the two of you against the problem, not against each other. You're a team, tackling shame, crappy socialization, gender norms, defensiveness, and all the other monsters that hide under the bed. Remind each other of that during the repair process. Sometimes simply saying, "Can we be on the same team?" can help you feel closer again.

Aim for Understanding, Not Agreement

Talking about sex is hard, and you and your partner are not always going to see things in the same way. Here's one of the most important keys to resolving conflict in your relationship: differentiate between understanding and agreement. Most people think that the only way to get over a fight is to get on the same page about it. You wind up in a tug-of-war, battling over who gets to be "right" and who gets to be "wrong" in the argument. But good communication doesn't mean that you're going to agree all the time. In fact, you're probably going to disagree more often than you agree. Instead, the goal of communication should be understanding.

One of the most shocking things I've learned in my time as a couples therapist is that two people can experience the exact same event in completely different ways. I can't tell you how many times I've done a session with a couple and thought, "Were these two people even in the same room? Did one of them hallucinate? Have they been body-snatched?" But that's just how life goes. You're filtering the world through your own set of lenses, and your partner is filtering the world through theirs. Both your experiences are valid. Even if it drives you bonkers, it's important to honor that your partner is having their own, unique experience.

What happened between Himari and Johan is the perfect example. For her birthday, Johan bought Himari expensive lingerie. Himari was extremely self-conscious about her body and hated lingerie, so the gift upset her. Johan had spent a lot of time and money on the gift, and he got upset that Himari was upset. They got into an enormous argument over a friggin' garter belt. I helped them understand that Himari didn't need to agree that the lingerie was a fabulous present, and Johan didn't need to agree that it was a cruel present. Instead, Himari needed to understand that Johan's intentions were good, and Johan needed to understand that the impact of his action was painful to Himari. The difference between intent and impact is so important. Johan's intentions with his gift were pure, and it hurt him that the impact was so painful to Himari. But that's just one of the realities of relationships. The intents that we have don't always create the impacts we wanted. Sometimes simply acknowledging that frustrating reality can help. You can say to each other, "My intent was X. I'm so sorry that the impact was Y."

The differences between intent and impact, and between understanding and agreement, are incredibly powerful. Perfect agreement is rare in any relationship, but understanding is almost always attainable. So, focus on validating each other's experiences. Remember that both your experiences are right and true, simply because you had them. There's space for both of you! Say things like "I understand how you feel that way" or "That makes sense to me" (even if it's a huge struggle for you!). Validating your partner's emotions will help them feel they have been deeply seen and heard. It tells them that their experience is real, and it's something that matters to you.

How to Apologize Without Losing Yourself

When it comes to apologies, I think about that old saying, "You can be right or you can be happy." I *love* being right, so sometimes it's *really* freakin' hard for me to apologize! It's especially hard to say sorry if you feel that your intent was good and you didn't mean to hurt your partner. But apologies are just so necessary in relationships. Nothing is more healing than hearing the words "I'm sorry" spoken with sincerity. Apology expert Harriet Lerner says that an apology is actually three gifts in one:

- A gift to the person you hurt, because it validates their experience when you take responsibility for your words and actions.
- A gift to yourself, because it gives you the opportunity to develop more emotional maturity.
- A gift to the relationship, because it gives you and your partner the faith that you can repair the harm you cause each other.

Even if you think you were right, even if your intentions were pure, apologize to your partner for the fight and for the impact your actions had on them.

Let It Go. Seriously.

Once you've had a proper conversation about a particular incident, don't bring it up again. Couples often dredge up the past because humans love looking for patterns. You get angry at your partner for playing a video game instead of coming to bed, and all of a sudden you're arguing about all the other times they prioritized their hobbies over intimacy. Your brain is like, "Ah, look, this thing is like that thing! Let's talk about that thing again! Oh, and it's like this thing, too! And like this one! Let's talk about *all the things!*" But this is exhausting and demoralizing, and it prevents any real progress from being made. Once it's resolved, it's over.

Make a Plan for Next Time

I like wrapping things up by addressing what I've learned from an argument and what I can do differently next time. Maybe you realize you can be a better communicator if your partner starts the conversation by saying, "I love you." That's a simple technique you could try going forward. Even if it's something that seems simple or even obvious, like "Next time I'm going to try harder to stay calm," that still helps you and your partner feel like there's progress in your relationship. Here are a few questions to ask yourselves:

"What is there to learn from this?"

"What do I understand about you better now?"

"What have I discovered about myself?"

"What can we do differently next time?"

Reconnect

Finally, try to reconnect with your partner by showing them love in some way. This is different for everyone, so ask your partner what makes them feel close to you again after an argument. Maybe it's taking a few minutes apart, going on a walk together, or repeating an inside joke. Xander's favorite thing is a good, old-fashioned hug. I like (and highly recommend) thanking each other for being willing to have tough conversations. You can even come up with a reconnection ritual that you do every time after a conflict. The point is just to do something that helps you both feel good.

To bring your *Sex Talks* adventure home, let's wrap up with a discussion about ways to continue prioritizing the twin flames of emotional and physical intimacy.

CHAPTER 11

MAKING SEX
A PRIORITY

OVER THE COURSE of your relationship, you will continue to feel the effects of the Fucking Fairy Tale. It will sing its siren song to you: "True love and hot sex should come *naturally*!" You'll get scared and paralyzed, and you won't want to put effort into your sex life. You'll feel the power of inertia telling you, "It's already been a week since you last had sex. What's one more night?" You'll feel too self-conscious or awkward to give feedback, make a request, or focus on your own pleasure.

Your sex life is going to need you to step up and protect it, over and over again. This is going to feel sad, frustrating, and downright exhausting at times. But your love and your intimacy deserve this active and ongoing effort.

Let's go back to my friend Francesca, who is desperate to keep her marriage alive. She and Jake are in a tough place, but they also love each other deeply and they don't want to give up. Here are some of the tools that I give her.

"I already know you're going to tell me to schedule it," Francesca groans.

"You bet your ass I am," I respond with a chuckle.

Believe me, I know that scheduling sex sounds terrible. It feels like something only maniacally type-A housewives do in a bad TV sitcom. (You know, with the huge family calendar on the wall and a color-coded sticker for the once-a-week sex date?) And I'll admit, when I first heard the idea of scheduled sex, I hated it. It felt like admitting defeat. I told myself I would never have a sex life that was so bad that I *had* to schedule it.

"Let me ask you this first," I tell Francesca. "If you don't put something on your calendar, how likely is it to happen?"

She snorts. "Zero chance."

"Exactly! Like with the kids, for example. If they come home and tell you they're in the school play next month, what are you going to do?"

"Put it on the calendar."

"Why?"

"Because it's important to me to be there, and I want to make sure we don't schedule anything else at that time."

"You're not going to say, 'No need to put it on the calendar; let's just see what happens. Maybe I'll show up, maybe I won't. If it's meant to be, it will happen.'"

She playfully rolls her eyes at me. "Of course not."

"And you're not going to judge yourself for putting it on the calendar, right? You're not going to think, *I must really not love my kids if I have to schedule showing up for them.*"

"Do you even want me to respond to that?" Francesca asks.

"Not really," I continue, picking up steam. "Look, we schedule the things that are important to us. Why should quality time with Jake be any different?"

Francesca takes a deep breath.

"Even when you have a great sex life, there are still so many other things fighting for your time and attention on a daily basis. You have to be purposeful about carving out time for each other and for intimacy, otherwise it won't happen."

I can tell that I'm getting close, but I haven't fully convinced Francesca yet. She tells me, "Scheduling it feels so clinical. I know I'm not supposed to say this, but I just wish it could feel more spontaneous. Or at least natural. And no, I don't feel that way about scheduling things with the kids, so don't even ask."

"Okay," I respond. "I want you to be brutally honest with me: Has spontaneity been working for you? Because I know you've been trying hard to have a spontaneous sex life for years. So, do you frequently feel the natural desire for sex at the exact same time that Jake feels it, and do you both magically have the time, space, privacy, and energy to be intimate in that moment?"

Francesca gives me a loving glare. I assume you're having the same reaction, dear reader. I don't think you'd have picked up this book if spontaneity has been working for you.

"I need to let you in on a little secret," I tell her. "You and Jake never really had a spontaneous sex life, even at the beginning of your relationship. When you first started dating, your entire relationship was foreplay. You were planning dates—dare I say *scheduling* dates—and you had days or even weeks at a time when you were building anticipation for seeing each other again. Remember how much time you would spend thinking about and getting ready for your dates? You were staying in contact, flirting constantly. There was nothing 'spontaneous' about any of that!"

"Ugh," Francesca says, not quite ready to give in. "But in the first year of our relationship, past the dating stage, it *did* feel spontaneous. No one ever initiated sex; it just happened."

"Yes, you did have all those early-relationship neurotransmitters working in your favor, but there was still a lot of effort involved, Babe. You were on your best behavior with each other, you were building intimacy, you were having lots of nonsexual touch, and you were actively seducing each other between your sexual escapades."

Francesca doesn't say anything.

"Holding out for spontaneous sex is a way of avoiding responsibility for your sex life. It's like waiting for Publishers Clearing House to show up at your door with a big check instead of looking for a higher-paying job, or hoping your partner will magically make the exact meal you're craving without your even mentioning that you're hungry."

She's tearing up a bit, so I give her a hug. "I get it. There are days when I wish my sex life with Xander was easy and spontaneous. But I know that most great things in life require at least a little effort, and I value myself, him, and our love enough to work for it. I know you feel the same about Jake."

"Okay," Francesca says, "you got me. I'll schedule my freakin' sex life."

"I'll tell you how to make it fun!" I assure her. "It's not going to feel clinical, I promise."

How to Plan for Sex—the Right Way

Scheduling sex definitely can feel clinical, but not if you set it up properly.

Notice that I keep using the word "plan"? Some people hate the word "scheduling," but a simple word swap can make all the difference. Say that you're planning for sex, or call it a date night instead, or a funny name like Sunday Funday or Afternoon Delight. That's an easy way to make it feel like a special inside joke rather than an obligation.

"I guess my biggest objection is what if I'm not in the mood when the day rolls around?" Francesca asks. "I worry about feeling pressured, like I can't say no."

"That's the beauty of the Easy Win," I tell her. "Pick one physical activity that you're always willing to do with love, no matter what else happened that day. It has to involve some form of physical contact, but it should be something simple, like cuddling or kissing. When you schedule sex, you're only agreeing to do your Easy Win activity. If you end up feeling like doing more in the moment, that's fine, but there's no pressure to do anything more than that. In the past, Xander and I said that we would keep the other company while they masturbate. So, if Xander is in the mood on our date night but I'm not, I can rest easy knowing that he'll take care of himself."

"Ooh, that's good," says Francesca. "If I know I don't have to do anything with my body, I could happily lie there with him. Maybe caress his chest or kiss his neck a little if I'm into it."

"Also, you're not signing a contract when you plan for sex," I tell her. "You and Jake are reasonable and empathetic people. You're not going to force each other to have sex if one of you is sick or in a terrible mood. Xander and I give each other veto power. If I'm canceling a sex date, my responsibility is to state that to him clearly ahead of time, and tell him why. I make space for him to be disappointed. And I have forty-eight hours to initiate a make-up date. You can change that timeline in your relationship, but it's nice to have some sort of arrangement like that."

Another fun idea is to take turns setting up your dates. You now know some of the things that help your partner feel open to intimacy. For example, maybe they love having ten minutes of alone time or a relaxing foot massage. When it's your turn to be in charge, do your best to get all those elements in place. Taking turns in this way helps you each feel cared for and seduced.

My recommendation is for you and your partner to talk openly about making a plan for sex, but you do have the option to keep that information for yourself. I've worked with some clients who are such planners that it helps them to know the specific days they're going to be intimate beforehand. They haven't explicitly set up a scheduled sex arrangement with their partner, but they take the initiative on the days they've committed to themselves.

The Other Half with Xander: Schedule Other Intimacy, Too

Given how hard it is to make the time for sex, it shouldn't come as a surprise that most couples struggle to carve out any sort of quality time for each other. Did you know that the average couple spends only thirty-five minutes per week having face-to-face conversations with each other? Yup, that's thirty-five minutes per *week* (not per day)! So, that's why we think it's just as important to schedule quality time together as it is to schedule sex. Plan date nights out, new activities, taking a walk around the neighborhood, other forms of physical touch, or just alone time together. You don't even have to leave the house if that's too complicated! The key is to just get it on the calendar, and then treat it as sacred time.

Scheduling quality time can also be a great way to continue getting more comfortable with the idea of scheduling sex. You get used to reserving time for each other. Most of us enjoy scheduling date nights, so see if you can bring that same energy to scheduled sexy nights, too!

How Often You Should Be Having Sex

Francesca asked me the question that couples inevitably have whenever I talk about scheduling sex: "What's a healthy amount of sex for a couple to have?" She's not alone in wondering; this is one of the most common questions I get asked. So, here's the exact number of times you should have sex per week . . .

Just kidding! There is no magic number that works for every couple. I've worked with couples who had sex multiple times a day and were miserable and unsatisfied, and I've worked with couples who had sex a few times a year and felt happy and connected.

We recently conducted a sexual frequency and satisfaction survey with our internet audience and received thirty-five thousand detailed responses. The top three response categories varied by less than 1 percent. That is, there was a nearly dead-even split among two to three times a month, once a week, and two to three times a week. We broke the responses down by age group and by whether or not the couple had kids, but there were no glaring differences then, either. (So much for the belief that getting older or having kids kills your sex life!) No matter the sexual frequency each survey responder indicated, the majority reported wanting to have more sex than they are currently having.

It's easy to get hyper-fixated on frequency because sex can feel like such a big, overwhelming topic. We want to focus on something that seems straightforward and quantifiable, like a number. But as I've already covered, it's way more useful to focus on the *quality* of sex rather than the *quantity*. Once you're having high-quality sex that's actually worth craving, the quantity typically falls into place, thanks to the enjoyment-desire connection. But on the other hand, if you force yourself to have sex when you're not in the mood just to reach a "healthy" quota, you're increasing the chances you'll have less enjoyable sex and will wind up craving it even less—the White Toast Problem.

After we got through the scheduling and frequency conversation, I shared a number of other quick tips with Francesca, so she could have plenty of tools in her tool kit.

Break Dry Spells as Quickly as Possible

Life is going to throw curveballs your way, and you are going to find yourself stuck in dry spells from time to time. That's normal, but try to get back in the saddle as quickly as possible. There's a funny kind of inertia when it comes to sex. If you forgot the concept of inertia from high school science, it's "An object at rest tends to stay at rest. An object in motion tends to stay in motion." The longer you go without having sex, the easier it feels to just keep not having sex.

A dry spell can feel embarrassing, so the mistake most couples make is to ignore it. But burying your head in the sand serves only to make the dry spell go on for longer and feel even worse. Instead, remember the importance of the Acknowledgment conversation (Chapter 5)! Say something like, "I know life has thrown a lot at us lately, but I'm really missing you and want to get back to a place of being more connected." Focus on the *emotions*, not on how long it's been since you last saw each other naked. This helps your partner recognize this is about connection, not about hitting a magic number.

Fortunately, inertia can work the other way, too. The more sex you have, the easier it feels to keep having sex. (That's why, ironically, couples who schedule sex often wind up having more non-scheduled sex, too.)

Fuck First

Dan Savage, host of *Savage Lovecast*, came up with this idea, which he defined as having sex *before* you go out to a fancy dinner date or big party, rather than waiting until you get home at the end of the night.[1] If I eat a big meal, the likelihood of my wanting to have sex afterward is extremely low. Have you ever tried to wriggle your way into tight, strappy lingerie when your belly is distended? Have you ever gotten the dreaded "whiskey dick" after one too many cocktails? Have you ever desperately tried to hold back a three-course-meal-induced fart while your partner was going down on you? If so, then you would benefit from fucking first!

Xander and I have expanded the Fuck First rule to mean prioritizing sex as early in the day as possible. Most couples leave sex until the very end of the evening. But by the time you're getting into bed, you're likely exhausted beyond belief. It's a really tough time to get excited about having sex. Intimacy is so much better when you actually have the energy for it. Obviously, the logistics may be trickier or not always possible depending on individual circumstances, but whenever you can, try to Fuck First. That might mean morning sex, an afternoon delight, letting the kids watch TV while you lock yourselves in the bathroom, or asking the babysitter to take the kids to the park—"So they don't get upset watching us leave!"

Explore

There's an endless world in front of you. Try new methods for keeping the Sex Drive Simmer alive, new forms of sexual and nonsexual touch, new ways of initiating. Try new foreplay techniques and bring back the old moves you haven't done in a while. Keep exploring in the bedroom together. Just do it. (And each other.)

Think and Talk About Sex Every Day

When Xander joined my business, he stayed behind the scenes for a couple years, focusing on the operational side of things. I kept telling him how valuable it would be for our community to hear from him, too, but he fended off my requests, insisting he didn't have anything valuable to add since he didn't have any training in human sexuality or psychotherapy.

In the shitshow that was 2020, I finally convinced him to join me on Instagram, YouTube, and our podcast *Pillow Talks*. We shared stories of our worst sexual failings. (Forgetting that I had a tampon in during sex, getting it impossibly stuck, and needing Xander to fish it out of me definitely ranks at the top of my most mortifying life moments.) We acted out (fully clothed) the worst sex positions we could find on the internet. We gave our audience ideas for how to talk dirty, how to ride Cowgirl, and how to politely ask their partner to tidy up their pubic hair before oral sex. We had a lot of fun goofing around together, but we also started to notice that our already great sex life was turning into something truly spectacular.

We were having *way* more sex. We were feeling more present with each other, like we were in our own little sex world, population two. We were having orgasms that were so insanely good they left us breathless, giddy, profoundly connected, and too dumbstruck to cobble together a full sentence.

We fully attribute the change to the fact that we were talking about sex openly and honestly every single day. (Aside from the aforementioned dumbstruck moments.) Even on the days we weren't having sex, that communication created a thread of connection between the two of us. The transformation was so noticeable that it drove us to write *Sex Talks*.

There's something truly special that happens when you talk about sex every day. The shame and embarrassment slowly peel away, and sex becomes a normal and natural part of your life—as it should be. Sex stays top of mind, and you find yourself wanting to seek out that connection with your partner more often. All the things that used to feel so awkward now feel lighter—even downright funny at times. Whether it's by taking turns reading this book to each other, asking each other one random sex-related question every evening, or watching Xander's and my Instagram stories together, challenge yourselves to talk about sex on a daily basis.

CHAPTER 12

FALLING BACK IN LOVE, FOR THE REST OF YOUR LIFE

WHENEVER YOU GET prescribed a course of antibiotics, your doctor tells you to take each and every dose. So many people start taking the medication, begin to feel better, then think they've made a full recovery. They stop taking their meds, and of course, they wind up getting sick again.

Just because your intimacy is in a good place now, that doesn't mean you stop doing the things that got it there. Keep putting effort into your emotional and physical intimacy. Keep reviewing and updating your User Manual, and share the latest version with each other. Keep your foot on the gas pedal. Keep adding logs to the fire. Keep watering your grass. This gets exhausting sometimes, I know, but your relationship deserves it.

Call me a sucker for love, but it pains me too much to see solid partnerships end because the couple didn't nurture their connection. Whenever I start working with a new couple, I tell them that I have three clients: each individual, plus the relationship. I encourage you to view your partnership as its own entity, and to be thoughtful about what it needs to thrive. You wouldn't blame a plant for dying if no one watered it, right? Your relationship is the same.

To wrap up your *Sex Talks* adventure, I'm opening my tool kit again and sharing some of my favorite ways to nurture your relationship and deepen your connection. There are a lot of techniques in this chapter because I'm thinking about my friend Emmy, who asked for a separation as I wrote this book. I know it's not my responsibility to save every (or any) relationship, and I know not every relationship is worth saving. But I love Emmy and Theo, and this one stings, so maybe I'm overextending myself a bit right now. I'm imagining that you and I are sitting down for tea the way Emmy and I do, and you're asking me to tell you how to keep your love alive. I tell you, "I don't just want to teach you how to give your relationship CPR and bring it back from the brink of death. I want to give you the tools to feel like you're falling back in love with each other, over and over again."

Identify Your Needle-Movers

We've covered a lot of ground in this book, and we're covering even more with the tips in this chapter. Once you've given everything a shot, identify the three things that had the biggest impact on your relationship. None of us has an unlimited amount of time, so we need to identify the specific techniques that give us the biggest bang for our buck.

Set Intentions

Start every morning asking yourself, "What could I do to give my partner and our relationship my best today?" Can you imagine what your relationship would be like if you did this?

The Other Half with Xander: Greet Each Other

My personal favorite trick is small, but shockingly effective: consciously acknowledge your partner's presence! Say proper Hellos and Goodbyes. Even when you're both already at home, look up from your phone, computer, or TV and make eye contact with your partner when they enter the room. Smile, and say Hi. You may already be rolling your eyes, but be honest with me: When was the last time you greeted your partner with genuine excitement?

The unfortunate reality is that it's so much easier *not* to acknowledge Vanessa's presence when she enters the room. Usually, I'm already in the middle of something and don't make immediate eye contact if she starts talking to me, as if she's a roommate I'm merely sharing space with. But if I think about it from the perspective of just how much I love Vanessa, then it feels really strange and cold to not even acknowledge her presence. Plus, every time you don't acknowledge your partner's presence, you're missing a potential opportunity for connection!

Vanessa was actually the one who pioneered this technique in our relationship. I'll never forget the first time she tried to intentionally acknowledge me. She was lying in bed, reading a book, while I was still brushing my teeth in the bathroom. As I walked back into the bedroom, she put her book down, made eye contact, gave me a big smile, and said, "Hey, Babe!" I was surprised, and looked around, as if she must be talking to someone else. But it felt so good!

Now we both jump on those tiny moments of connection. It just takes a few seconds to acknowledge each other, but it makes us both smile and feel loved multiple times a day.

Ask Better Questions

Tell me how many times you've had this conversation:

> "How was your day?"
> "Fine. How was yours?"
> "Fine. How was yours?"
> "Fine. How was . . . wait, I already responded."

When Xander and I first met, we would spend hours talking about everything and nothing, but as the years marched on, those kinds of conversations started to feel harder to come by. Instead, we started having plenty of transactional discussions about schedules or the weather, and longer and longer stretches of silence.

Here's what we eventually discovered: if you want to get that conversational spark back, you have to ask each other better questions and make space for more thoughtful responses. Here are some interesting options:

> "What initially attracted you to me?"
> "What made you fall in love with me?"
> "When do you feel the closest or most connected to me?"
> "What are the strengths of our relationship?"
> "When do you find me the most attractive?"
> "What are our core values as a couple?"
> "What's something you love about me today?"

Create Rituals

One of the best things about being in a relationship is having rituals that feel unique to your relationship. Rituals are things that the two of you do together on a regular basis that feel special, celebratory, and/or romantic. They make you feel like you're in a top-secret club.

For example, Xander and I had so much fun on our honeymoon that we decided one wasn't enough. Instead, we created a ritual whereby we take a trip for our anniversary every year. It has become one of our favorite ways to celebrate our love, and we both look forward to it every year.

Another ritual we have is taking our two pugs, Winston and Maggie, on a walk together every single day. It would be easy to think of walking the dogs as a chore that one of us is responsible for, but since we started thinking of it as a ritual that we do together, it has become so much more enjoyable. It's our time to get some fresh air, clear our heads, talk about our days in more meaningful ways, and see new parts of our neighborhood.

Here are some other ideas for rituals you can create:

- Say three things you're grateful for about your relationship before you go to bed every night.
- Read a new book together every month.
- If you're married, watch your wedding video together, or reread your vows to each other, every year on your anniversary. If you're not married, rehash the story of the day you met.
- Decide to volunteer together during the holidays every year.
- Spend five minutes together over your morning coffee.
- Cook a meal together once a week.
- Make out with each other for at least a few seconds every time you leave for the day or go to bed at night.

Actually Have Date Nights

You already know you should have date nights. But do you have them? For most couples these days, "quality time" means sitting on opposite ends of the couch, watching TV while you also fold laundry and scroll through Facebook. I hate to break it to you, but this does not count as quality time!

Date night sounds trite, but it's absolutely essential to the health of any relationship. You need time for just the two of you, without any sort of distractions. You need to have fun together. You need to be reminded of those early days in your relationship when you were so fascinated by each other that you couldn't possibly imagine wanting to do anything else other than bask in the presence of your partner.

In particular, I recommend trying to do new things on your date nights. Going out to dinner can be nice, but you've probably had hundreds of dinner dates together. Instead, push yourselves out of your comfort zones and try something a bit more off the beaten path every once in a while. Google "creative date ideas" or the town or city that you live in plus the phrase "date night ideas."

Check in Regularly

This is such a simple suggestion, but it's a powerful one that hardly any couples do: have regular "State of Our Union" relationship check-ins. We have regular check-ins with our doctor, with our tax guy, with our kid's teacher, but so few of us make the time for a check-in with our partner. We get so caught up in our endless to-do lists and daily anxieties that we feel like the only option is to *just keep moving*. But taking the time to stop, look back, honestly evaluate what you've done, and brainstorm how you can improve in the next round, can transform your relationships. Check-ins give you the chance to be grateful, to celebrate accomplishments, and to be intentional about becoming a better person and partner.

Depending on what works best for your relationship, you can do daily, weekly, and/or monthly check-ins with your partner. During your check-in, ask each other these kinds of questions:

"What did we do really well today/this week/this month?"

"When did you feel closest to me today/this week/this month?"

"What are you grateful for?"

"What challenged us?"

"What do we need more or less of in the next week/month?"

"How can we be the best possible partners to each other in the next week/month?"

The Attitude of Gratitude

There are few things more capable of transforming your relationship than gratitude. It's so easy to take your partner for granted, and to forget about all the little ways they show you their love and affection. We're quick to focus on the fact that they left yet another cup directly on top of the dishwasher instead of putting it *inside*, and neglect to see that they wiped down every surface in the entire kitchen. Yes, you and your partner are working toward a more intimate relationship, but you already have so much to be grateful for. Make an extra effort to acknowledge and appreciate each other for the things you already do.

I'll be honest: a lot of the couples I work with roll their eyes at the notion of gratitude. It sounds a little cheesy or juvenile. But research done by the University of Georgia found that gratitude is "the most consistent significant predictor of marital quality."[1]

The good news is that it's ridiculously easy to show appreciation to your partner, and even one simple sentence can feel so good for both of you! I can't think of many other things that have such a high payoff for so little effort. Every time you notice something that your partner has done for you, say thank you. You won't believe how much you can light your partner up by saying something as simple as "Hey, I really appreciate that you took out that stinky trash." Sometimes I like getting into a goofy mood with this one and going overboard. "Xander, I'm so thankful that you made the bed this morning! . . . Do you know how loved I feel when I see that you put your boxers in the laundry hamper? . . . And have I mentioned how glorious it is to see the towels put away? You're the best!" I can be talking about the stupidest, most insignificant tasks, but he still gets giddy with pride.

I also like starting and ending every day with a few seconds of gratitude. In the morning I think about specific moments from the previous day that I'm grateful for, like Xander bringing me a freshly brewed cup of tea. In the evenings, we share our gratitude with each other.

And don't forget to specifically call out the new things your partner is trying, thanks to your Sex Talks. Positive reinforcement of the behaviors you want to keep seeing works so much better than criticism of the behaviors you hate. The more seen and valued your partner feels for their new action steps, the more likely they are to do them. So, tell them, "It's so freaking hot when you initiate sex with a dirty text message," and watch the naughty texts keep flowing.

Keep Being Vulnerable

I've spent more than two hundred pages making the case that communication is the key to a smoking-hot sex life. But there's one other variable that's just as important—vulnerability. Lemme get all Brené Brown on your ass and remind you that "there is no intimacy without vulnerability."[2]

Intimacy isn't about having the Fucking Fairy Tale version of sex or love. Real intimacy is about making the choice to be vulnerable, over and over again. It's about choosing to ask for power play, even when it's easier to pretend you're happy with vanilla sex. It's about choosing to initiate, even though you got turned down the day before. It's about choosing to let your partner see your tears instead of turning away. It's about choosing to have the tough conversation, even when you'd rather plug your ears and hum to yourself. It's about choosing to show up for yourself, your partner, and your love, every single day.

DON'T STOP!

I HAVE TO make a confession. As much as I love talking about extraordinary sex lives and relationships, sometimes I catch myself feeling pessimistic about our collective capacity to create that kind of change. I hear an awful lot of stories about people being jerks to each other in the bedroom. My brain can leap to justifications that it's because of the lack of honest and informative conversations about sex. But sometimes my heart just feels heavy, and I find myself wondering, "Is there any hope?" Most therapists deal with compassion fatigue from time to time, and I'm certainly no exception.

One of the couples from Conversation 4 (Chapter 8) is the prime example. Remember the woman who said her husband "doesn't feel like taking the time" to make sure she orgasms because she "takes way more effort"? Let me tell you the full story of what happened with this couple. We'll call her April.

April had originally sent this message to us via Instagram. I distinctly remember reading her DM to Xander, and saying, "This guy sucks. It's so toxic and unhelpful when people get into scorekeeping mode with their partner. And he seems selfish and unreasonable. Who cares if it takes her a few more minutes to have a good time?"

I was feeling spicy that day, so I wrote back to April, "I would tell him: 'I don't feel like letting *you* come 75 percent of the time,' and see how he feels about that. This is an unacceptable attitude for him to have. If he doesn't care enough about you having a good experience, he doesn't deserve access to your body."

April responded right away, saying, "It's the worst. He has also said a lot of negative things about going down on me, which has made me feel so insecure. It was out of character because he's a wonderful guy and I was surprised to hear all those things. I wonder if maybe he feels inadequate so he just doesn't want to go there and feels defensive about it? As frustrating as it all is, I don't want to be brash about any of it. Do you have any advice on how I could make it seem less daunting to him? I'll try anything."

I will fully admit that I felt jaded about the future for these two. What on earth could I do to help this man if he didn't think that his wife was deserving of the same experience he got to have in the bedroom? How could I convince him to stop being a lazy tool and "feel like taking the time" to pleasure her? I wanted to give up, but Xander reminded me that there are a lot of couples in our audience going through the same sorts of things, so we decided to do a story on Instagram about this couple. With April's permission, we anonymously shared the details of her story.

I kicked us off by saying, "It really bums me out that not only is this woman having a bad experience with sex, but she's also having to take on the emotional labor of figuring out how to help him be a better partner."

Xander jumped in and added, "Let's try to throw this guy a bone for a second. He may be missing some key information about how sex and female orgasm work. For example, that penetration alone is not the most pleasurable activity for the vast majority of vulva owners, whereas it is for most penis owners. So, it's no wonder that he's able to come so much quicker than she can. She just needs more time and the proper stimulation."

I agreed with Xander rationally, but my heart was still angry for April, so I said, "This tit-for-tat attitude that he has around sex is unhelpful and unkind. Sex is an act that we do *together*, and you both deserve to have a pleasurable experience. Sex isn't great because you both got exactly five minutes of attention. Sex is great because you both experienced pleasure! Who cares exactly how long or exactly how much effort you took to get there."

I took a deep breath before continuing. "What I would say to this husband is: 'It doesn't matter that it takes me more time or more effort. What matters is the end result. It's important to me that you have a good experience, and it should be important to you that I have a good experience. I want to be a team in this rather than keeping score.'" Giving specific communication scripts always calms me, so I got another idea in the moment. "This woman insists that this was out of character for her husband, so she could disarm him right away by saying something like 'I know you're a good man. I know that you care about me and my experience. I don't think you realize how unkind and uncaring your words are coming off, so I want us to try having this conversation again.'"

I wrapped it up with, "If you're a woman and you find yourself feeling self-conscious about taking too much time or effort with your male partner, first of all, it's probably because the way that you're having sex is prioritizing his pleasure, not your own. But the bottom line is that you deserve to have sex that's *for you*, that feels good, and safe, and is an enjoyable experience."

April responded immediately, and said, "This was great! I'll ask those big questions and take it from there. I think the hardest thing about having sex is having conversations about it. Our recent conversation was the first time I had brought it up in a really long time, so I feel encouraged to keep that conversation going."

My pessimism wasn't assuaged in the slightest. I just felt sad for her for having to do so much work.

But lo and behold, a few weeks later I got another message from April. She wrote: "Things have been *so* much better with my husband. Talking about the fact that I wasn't orgasming was challenging and made intimacy weird for a bit. But I think he needed to work through feeling discouraged and ashamed that my pleasure wasn't magically aligning with his before understanding what needed to change. Also worth noting that 90 percent of what we knew about sex going into marriage was learned from porn. Which is obviously far from educational when it comes to female orgasm! He's now prioritizing my pleasure, and we're having a great time together. It's a night-and-day difference. Getting the guts to keep advocating for myself really played a crucial part in this, so thank you for the push to keep talking about it!"

I was flooded with so many emotions as I read April's words. Gratitude toward her for reaching out with this unexpected update. Sadness about the damage I know that a porn-only sex education can cause. Genuine excitement that their sex life was undergoing a massive change. Shame for feeling so pessimistic and hopeless about their future. And a fuck-ton of inspiration to keep doing this work. Yes, this husband absolutely acted like a jerk toward his wife. And yet, he was still capable of taking some time, processing his thoughts and emotions, and becoming a better partner to her.

If you made it through to the end of this book, first, let me just say that you're a badass and I'm proud of you. Even if you read it on your own and haven't uttered a peep to your partner, you've still done something that most people don't have the courage to do. I know you're only going to keep developing a healthier and happier relationship with sex, and I'm so excited for what's in store for you.

And I also know that you may find yourself feeling pessimistic about the future of your relationship. Maybe your partner refused to read this book with you. Maybe you're worried about how they'll respond to you trying out some of the exercises and techniques. I know *Sex Talks* asks a *lot* of you and your partner. Sex and partnership ask a lot of us! Sometimes it feels easier to give in to our fears and not take any sort of action. To accept a lackluster or even straight-up shitty sex life rather than have the courage to open your mouth and start talking about it.

I get it! Obviously even I lose my faith at times. And I continue to struggle with sexual communication in my own relationship. Even after fourteen years together, and even after all of the progress we've made, Xander and I still had a handful of conversations for the first time *ever* in the course of writing this book. (The one about the rogue finger in the butt obviously being the most memorable.)

I needed April's story as a reminder that, in the depths of my being, I really and truly believe that all of us are capable of creating extraordinary sex lives. I know this is possible for you, too. Although the five conversations are now over, the journey doesn't end here. Keep being brave, keep talking about sex, and keep us up to date on how things go for you.

IDENTIFYING YOUR CONVERSATIONAL STARTING POINT

MOST COUPLES WILL benefit from all the Sex Talks in this book, so my recommendation is to go through them in order. But if you want to get a sense for which of the conversations will be most powerful for you, take this simple quiz!

WHAT ASPECT OF SEX FEELS MOST EMBARRASSING OR CHALLENGING TO YOU?

A. All of it! The whole topic feels taboo.

B. Intimacy as a whole. I struggle to open up and connect with another person.

C. Sex drive. I don't feel interested in sex very often.

D. Enjoying the experience. I don't get what all the fuss is about.

E. Breaking out of my routine.

WHAT TYPES OF COUPLES DO YOU FIND YOURSELF LOOKING UP TO THE MOST?

A. Couples who can talk about anything with each other.

B. Couples who seem to be deeply in love.

C. Couples who still desire each other, even after decades together.

D. Couples who have explosive orgasms.

E. Couples who are always trying something new.

WHEN THINGS ARE BAD IN YOUR SEX LIFE, WHAT STATEMENT DESCRIBES YOUR RELATIONSHIP THE BEST?

A. My partner and I don't talk about our sex life.

B. My partner and I feel disconnected from each other.

C. Either me or my partner (or both of us) have a hard time getting turned on.

D. The sex that we have feels one-sided.

E. We repeat the same sex routine over and over again.

WHAT DO YOU WISH YOUR PARTNER DID MORE OFTEN?

A. Talked to me about our relationship.

B. Did a better job making me feel loved and cared for.

C. Turned me on.

D. Focused on my pleasure and helped me feel good.

E. Suggested fun new things for us to try in the bedroom together.

WHAT'S YOUR MAIN GOAL FOR YOUR SEX LIFE?

A. Just to be able to talk about it openly.

B. To feel more emotionally connected to my partner.

C. To increase my libido and feel turned on more easily.

D. To have more pleasurable sex.

E. To get creative and experiment in the bedroom.

Mostly As: Start with Conversation 1—Acknowledgment

Mostly Bs: Start with Conversation 2—Connection

Mostly Cs: Start with Conversation 3—Desire

Mostly Ds: Start with Conversation 4—Pleasure

Mostly Es: Start with Conversation 5—Exploration

ACKNOWLEDGMENTS

AS A LIFELONG bookworm who spent an embarrassingly significant part of her childhood alone at the public library, I've always dreamed of writing a book of my own. That dream would not have been possible without some very special and important people, so I want to thank them with my whole heart.

Thank you to Xander for being the best possible partner in life and in this book; for never batting an eye when I asked you to try yet another weird sexperiment; for keeping me on my toes in our relationship and always giving me something new to write about; for making me laugh (usually with your dancing) even when the book-writing process got way harder than I ever thought it would; for inspiring me with your vulnerability; and, of course, for your wandering finger. I love you.

Thank you to my parents for being brave enough to whisper the word "sex" during that fateful car ride, and for now being so open that I'm often the one blushing. I love you both to the moon and back.

Thank you to all our friends and families for being so proud and supportive. Your love, laughter, and encouragement mean the world to me.

Special thanks to Richelle Fredson. This book would not exist without your brilliance. You have a special talent for pulling books out of people, my friend! To Wendy Sherman for believing in us right from the get-go, and for being a shark in the best possible way. To Michelle Herrera Mulligan:

your vision, guidance, and thoughtfulness shaped this book into something we didn't even realize was possible. Thank you to Sandi and the team at Hilsinger-Mendelson. Thank you to every single person at Simon & Schuster who touched this book. You all helped make it better, and I'm eternally grateful to you.

Thank you to our team at V+X. I love each and every one of you so much it makes my heart hurt. Thank you for reading early drafts, giving feedback, asking great questions, and sharing your own stories. Thank you for running the business so we could focus on the book. Thank you for letting me cry when I needed to cry and for making me laugh when I needed to laugh. You're the best.

Thank you to our community for being a part of this process every single step of the way. Thank you for answering our polls, giving us ideas for chapter titles, and sharing your most intimate stories.

And, finally, thank you to every person who has ever asked me a question about sex. It means a lot to me that you trusted me to be your guide. This book is for you, and I hope it brings more orgasms and more love into your life!

NOTES

Chapter 1: Destroying the Fucking Fairy Tale

1. Alyson Shapiro, John Gottman, and Sybil Carrère, "The Baby and the Marriage: Identifying Factors That Buffer Against Decline in Marital Satisfaction After the First Baby Arrives," *Journal of Family Psychology* 14, no. 1 (March 2020): 59–70, https://doi.org/10.1037/0893-3200.14.1.59.

Chapter 2: Creating Your User Manual

1. Emily Nagoski, *Come as You Are* (New York: Simon & Schuster, 2015).
2. Debby Herbenick, Vanessa Schick, Stephanie Sanders, Michael Reece, and J. Fortenberry, "Pain Experienced During Vaginal and Anal Intercourse with Other Sex Partners: Findings from a Nationally Representative Probability Study in the United States," *Journal of Sexual Medicine* 12, no. 4 (April 2015): 1040–51, https://doi.org/10.1111/jsm.12841.

Chapter 3: Setting Your Rules of Engagement

1. "National Intimate Partner and Sexual Violence Survey: 2015 Data Brief," Centers for Disease Control, accessed April 6, 2022, https://www.cdc.gov/violenceprevention/datasources/nisvs/2015NISVSdatabrief.html.
2. "Victims of Sexual Violence: Statistics," Rape, Abuse, and Incest National Network, accessed April 6, 2022, https://www.rainn.org/statistics/victims-sexual-violence.

Chapter 4: Building the Foundation for Your Sex Talks

1. Sybil Carrère and John Gottman, "Predicting Divorce among Newlyweds from the First Three Minutes of a Marital Conflict Discussion," *Family Process* 38, no. 3 (September 1999): 293–301, https://doi.org/10.1111/j.1545 5300.1999.00293.x.

Chapter 6: The Second Conversation: Connection

1. Gary Chapman, *The Five Love Languages* (Farmington Hills, MI: Walker Large Print, 2010).

2. Tyler Schmall, "Parents Get Way Less Than an Hour per Day of 'Me Time,'" *New York Post*, October 3, 2018, https://nypost.com/2018/10/03/parents-get -way-less-than-an-hour-per-day-of-me-time/.

3. Daniel Carlson, Amanda Miller, Sharon Sassler, and Sarah Hanson, "The Gendered Division of Housework and Couples' Sexual Relationships: A Reexamination," *Journal of Marriage and Family* 78, no. 4 (August 2016): 975–95, https://doi.org/10.1111/jomf.12313.

Chapter 7: The Third Conversation: Desire

1. Emily Impett and Letitia Peplau, "Sexual Compliance: Gender, Motivational, and Relationship Perspectives," *Journal of Sex Research* 40, no. 1 (2003): 87–100, https://doi.org/10.1080/00224490309552169.

Chapter 8: The Fourth Conversation: Pleasure

1. "National Survey of Sexual Health and Behavior: Key Findings," Indiana University, Bloomington, accessed April 6, 2022, https://nationalsexstudy .indiana.edu/keyfindings/index.html.

Chapter 10: What to Do When Conversations Go Off the Rails

1. Ibid.

Chapter 11: Making Sex a Priority

1. Dan Savage, "Should the Duggar Girls #FuckFirst?" *Stranger*, November 5, 2014, https://www.thestranger.com/seattle/should-the-duggar-girls-fuckfirst/Content?oid=20951878.

Chapter 12: Falling Back in Love, for the Rest of Your Life

1. Allen Barton, Ted Futris, and Robert Nielsen, "Linking Financial Distress to Marital Quality: The Intermediary Roles of Demand/Withdraw and Spousal Gratitude Expressions," *Journal of the International Association for Relationship Research* 22, no. 3 (September 2015): 536–49, https://doi.org/10.1111/pere.12094.

2. Brené Brown, *Daring Greatly: How the Courage to Be Vulnerable Transforms the Way We Live, Love, Parent, and Lead* (New York: Penguin, 2012).